inner chi
for energy
Rejuvenation & Longevity

inner chi
for energy
Rejuvenation & Longevity

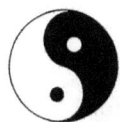

A T'ai Chi Sourcebook by

Virginia L. Harford

Inner Chi for Energy is a Sourcebook, an introduction, to encourage, motivate and inspire a person to check out the benefits of *T'ai Chi* or *Qigong* and some of the books, videos and other information that is available. It does not have specific *T'ai Chi* or *Qigong* movements. It does have two meditations to peak one's interest. A wealth of information is available. May the references in this book help you investigate some of the forms, benefits and well-being that the practice of *T'ai Chi* and *Qigong* will bring into your life!

The author of *Inner Chi for Energy* wishes the reader to know that the ideas and movements in this book are not intended as medical advice. Please consult your physician or trained health professional before adopting any of them.

ISBN: 978-1-929995-04-2
Second edition: 2015

Published by
Virginia L. Harford
e-mail: virginiah9@gmail.com

Book and cover design by: Patricia Garcia Arreola

Dedicated to
my students, teachers, and friends
from whom I have learned so much
and Justin Stone, Originator of *T'ai Chi Chih*

On the front cover is:
The Phoenix: The Icon of Rejuvenation

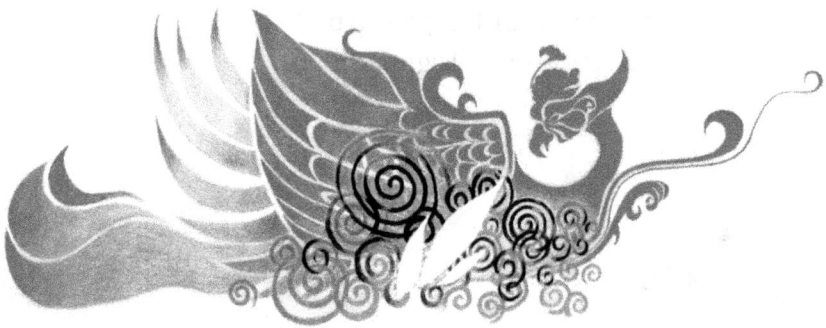

The Phoenix is considered the most beautiful bird in the world; it brings good fortune and it lives forever recreating itself. The awesome Phoenix has been in mythologies of cultures around the world from ancient times to the present.

The sketch of the Phoenix is by Robert Johnson, an artist in San Miguel de Allende, Guanajuato, Mexico.

Comments

"As a teacher of *Qi Gong* and a *Doctor of Oriental Medicine*, I highly recommend Virginia's latest book *Inner Chi for Energy—Rejuvenation and Longevity—A T'ai Chi Sourcebook*. She describes all of the amazing results one can experience in their own lives. Anyone with a regular practice will receive many health benefits."
> — Dr. Denise Gelpi Aughtman, D.O.M.

"While house/pet sitting in San Miguel de Allende, I was fortunate to be able to attend Virginia's *T'ai Chi* classes. I found it a great practice to ground and center myself, which resulted in my feeling more at peace, flexible and balanced. As the weeks went by, the movements became increasingly easy to flow with and eventually it was like a beautiful meditation. Over time, I am looking forward to achieving the many long-term benefits of *T'ai Chi.*"
> — Rose Kettner, Retired Nurse

"My Testimonial to *T'ai Chi*: I have found it very difficult to sit still and meditate for an hour. As soon as I realized that *T'ai Chi* was a MOVING meditation, I started to feel its benefits. After an hour of *T'ai Chi*, I feel both energized AND relaxed."
> — Judy Rosenthal, Ph.D.

Comments (continued)

"*T'ai Chi* is a calming exercise that leaves you feeling centered and invigorated. I found it helped my neuropathy, giving me better balance."
— Carol Turner

"I never discovered *T'ai Chi* until this year (2013). It has given me energy which was a surprise as this is a low-keyed exercise and is very peaceful and slow moving. When time passes without *T'ai Chi*, I can notice a difference in the way I feel during my day. There are many rewards for practicing *T'ai Chi*."
— June Beerman

"I met *T'ai Chi Chih* about 8 months ago thanks to Virginia Harford. I am discovering it to be many things. It is a lovely form of meditation—I have always liked walking meditation. Somehow it keeps my mind occupied, and *T'ai Chi* enables me to get into a meditative state without any problem. It enables me to stay much more focused throughout the day. Physically, it helps my ability to maintain balance and it strengthens my legs and arms. I suppose I must confess that for me, it is just fun to accomplish the movements gracefully and feel the tingling in my hands and fingers and even occasionally in my lower *tan t'ien*. As I practice more, I am able to come to a meditative state more quickly and stay there more easily. I can only thank Virginia for sharing this gift of peace with me."
— Sue Leonard, Nurse Practioner

Table of Contents

List of Research Articles: Benefits
of Doing *T'ai Chi* or *Gi Gong*

*The motion should be rooted in the feet, released
through the legs, controlled by the waist, and
manifested through the fingers.*
— Chang San-feng, 13th Century

T'ai Chi
Overview of Benefits

太极

T'ai Chi improves overall fitness, coordination, and agility. People who practice *T'ai Chi* on a regular basis tend to have good posture, flexibility, and range of motion, are more mentally alert, and sleep more soundly at night.

Consistent practice will improve one's health because the movements stimulate the circulatory, lymphatic and immune systems as well as the central nervous system. *T'ai Chi* circulates energy (*Chi*) through the meridians. The strength of the bones and muscles and the functions of the metabolic, respiratory and cardiovascular systems are greatly improved. It is especially good for people with a chronic illness, anxiety, viral infections, depression, or any stress-related conditions.

> "T'ai Chi is both a preventive and complementary therapy for a wide range of conditions. Specifically, it is beneficial for chronic pain, gout, heart disease, high blood pressure, arthritis, osteoporosis, diabetes, headaches, fibromyalgia, rheumatoid arthritis, osteoarthritis, and sleep disorders. The deep breathing of T'ai Chi regulates the respiratory system, helping to treat respiratory ailments such as asthma, bronchitis, and emphysema. It also stimulates

the abdomen, which aids digestion and helps relieve constipation and gastrointestinal conditions.

Many clinical studies indicate that elderly people who practice T'ai Chi have better hand eye coordination, and are much less prone to falls, both serious health risks to people in that age group."
— from a *T'ai Chi Overview*, the University of
Maryland Medical Center

To summarize: The benefits from practicing *T'ai Chi* are both physical and mental. Done regularly, *T'ai Chi* improves muscle tone, flexibility, balance, and coordination. Older people have discovered that it increases their energy and agility, sharpens their reflexes and they have an overall feeling of well-being. Some have used it for healing and as an addition to other programs for chronic conditions of arthritis, fibromyalgia or heart disease. Research has discovered that *T'ai Chi* often holds a person's interest longer than other types of exercise and it is safe for people of all ages and fitness abilities.

Lao Tzu in the Tao Te Ching talks about the power of gentleness and yielding:

When people are born, they are gentle and weak.
At death they are hard and stiff.
Green plants are pliant and tender while living.
When they're dead, they are withered and dried.
Therefore the stiff and unbending follow death.
The supple and yielding follow life.

Introduction by Oonah Perdue
(*T'ai Chi* Instructor Featured on PBS)

太极

My personal pursuit of beauty and serenity led me to embrace the practice of *T'ai Chi Chih* some years ago. Since then, I joyously have shared its treasures. It was my privilege to have learned these wonderful movements from their master, Justin Stone. He gave them to us from his deep knowledge of the more extensive, and thus more demanding, *T'ai Chi Chuan*.

Seijaku in Japanese means serenity in the midst of activity. The practice is simple; the result is profound. These ancient exercises were brought from China as a solution to the stress and health problems of the modern world.

Finding *T'ai Chi* brought together my upbringing in a medical family and my love for the Orient where I once lived as a British physician's wife. It was in China that I first was impressed with the graceful exercises done by so many people in public parks, although the disciplines then were unknown to me.

So it is with much interest and satisfaction that I have read Virginia Harford's book, a storehouse of knowledge you are about to enter. She has brought us practicality in understanding *T'ai Chi*, but she also has reached back to the Oriental ancients for the lore that will help us comprehend them. Her compilation here is greatly embellished by her activity in today's health and fitness field and supported by her knowledge of the arts, around the world travels, and life in the Orient.

Once you have read the book and begun the study of *T'ai Chi*, I hope you will find, as I have, that practice of these calming and tranquil exercises is an experience, one that sends you on a journey into happiness and marks your return with an abundance of well-being and marvelous energy.

Background:

With a natural interest in health due to her family background in England, Oonagh began exploring ways to improve one's health. While living in China during World War II, she saw a large segment of the population practicing *T'ai Chi Chuan* daily to prevent aging. In 1975, Oonagh Perdue became a *T'ai Chi Chih* instructor, certified by Justin Stone.

From 1976, Oonah Perdue had taught *T'ai Chi Chih* classes and seminars for colleges, corporations, resorts and health facilities throughout the United States. She also taught classes at Arizona State University, Phoenix College and Rio Salado Community College. She was featured in a PBS documentary, "The Dragon and the Eagle," broadcast on television stations during 1991.

(Oonagh Perdue was a friend who passed away in November of 2011. She was born in October of 1912 so she was 101 years old. She often said to me that *T'ai Chi Chih* was "youthifying". Thank you Oonagh for great inspiration.)

Foreword

大极

Do you want to have more energy?
Do you desire to lose weight?
Do you want to look younger and live longer?
Do you want to cope with stress?
Do you want to have more joy in your life?
Do you want a gentle health regime?
Do you want to learn one of the great secrets in life?

Doing *T'ai Chi* movements may be your answer. I want to share my love of doing *T'ai Chi* movements with you. It is one of the great secrets of circulating energy in your body. The wonderful gentle movements of *T'ai Chi* have dramatically improved my life. I had been in an automobile accident that resulted in devastating lower back pain for over a year. Every day because of the pain, I would become very fatigued in the afternoon. I began doing the *T'ai Chi* movements and other *Chi Kungs*.

While doing the movements, I would immediately feel my fingers tingling and energy going throughout my entire body. After several weeks, I found I didn't need as much sleep. Then a month into the regime, I no longer became exhausted in the middle of the afternoon. Several months later, my sense of smell became keener. I no longer had lower back pain!

OMG! After a whole year of having massage, biofeedback, heat packs, hypnosis, hot showers, etc., I finally felt so much better. I didn't have to have people go shopping for me anymore. I was not in the continual pain that was so enervating. At times, I would have to sit in a steno chair that had wheels to help me get around. The pain medicines the doctors would give me made me nauseated and I could not take them.

I felt the movements were so valuable and could help many people. I wanted to share them with others. It was the *T'ai Chi* that made the big difference for me. I took the *T'ai Chi Chih* Teacher Training in 1992 and started to teach classes. I was so intrigued that I learned a lot about the energy that is being generated throughout the body; *Chi* it is called. In yoga it is called *prana*. When my mother was dying and on Hospice, I did *T'ai Chi* movements every morning to help with my stress and anguish.

Much was written about the three *tan tiens* which store the *Chi*, and while doing the movements, the *Chi* is going through the meridian system of the body. It is the meridians in the body that acupuncture also addresses. These movements were kept secret for many centuries. They were practiced quietly in the temples of China and Tibet for thousands of years enabling the monks to live well over 100 years.

I was so enthusiastic, I also read a lot about the history. I have short quotes from ancient manuscripts that beautifully describe the movements and how to do them. *T'ai Chi* emphasizes slow movements and tranquility of mind. The underlying principle is that action follows thought. All internal exercises are controlled by such consciousness, so one must therefore be quiet and calm before beginning and then apply one's total concentration. Relaxation is all important.

Special attention is paid to balance; lightness and suppleness characterize the movements. They should be done slowly and smoothly as the motions are in accord with the natural movements of the body. The movements regenerate your body by working on the lymphatic system, thus stimulating the body's immunity. They also benefit the cardiovascular system for improved circulation.

I learned two systems of *Chi Kungs* (which means daily workout and the circulation of *Chi*). One of the systems was originated by Justin Stone. He had taught *T'ai Chi Chuan* and wanted to teach a different form not as demanding so he developed *T'ai Chi Chih*. There are estimated to being over 70,000 different *Chi Kungs*. Among them are the "T'ai Chi Ruler" and "The Swimming Dragon" to which I was also introduced and practiced.

After doing the movements of *T'ai Chi*, we were taught to practice the Microcosmic Orbit Meditation. It moves *Yin* (cool) energy up the spine cooling the body. The energy produced can be used for healing. In opening up this microcosmic channel, it is possible to breathe the life force energy up the spine.

Chi Gong only became popular in the People's Republic of China since 1982. It was ignored by the elite. Those that carried on the practice were Confucian scholars, Taoists, Buddhist priests and students of ancient medicine and martial arts. Those growing up during the Communist period did not know about it until 1979 when *Chi Gong* was brought to the attention of the general public.

Chi Gong had been rediscovered and a virtual craze went through China. It is estimated that in Beijing alone there are over three hundred thousand practitioners. There are two categories: hard and soft.

Hard *Chi Gong*, for example, is breaking steel rods with one's foot or splitting bricks by hand, or breaking a piece of marble by running into it head first. This became very common in China and many earned their living by doing this.

Soft *Chi Gong* was mastered to enable one to prevent or overcome illness and also to cure certain illnesses in others. The latter would be shifting energy from oneself to the patient. This often would take many years of *Chi Gong* practice, sometimes over ten or twenty, to build up the practitioner's energy. Western science, overall, ignores the nature and source of *Chi* energy. However, in some areas, acupuncture has become popular.

The Chinese believe that we need *chi* as we need blood. More than two thousand years ago in *The Yellow Emperor's Classic of Internal Medicine*, it was determined that there were two separate circulations in the body. One was the circulation of blood. This was thousands of years before William Harvey discovered this in England. The second was the circulation of *Chi*, an energy pumped by the lungs to circulate in invisible body tracts. This dual circulation theory of blood (*Yin*) and *Chi* (*Yang*) indicated the two were interrelated.

Until the 1980s, the existence of *Chi Gong* masters was considered to be a state secret in China. It had been practiced in China for over three thousand years and often it fell into obscurity. It was a political decision to have *Chi Gong* become familiar in order to help China's over one billion people and cure thousands of patients. Chinese scientists claim to have proved that *Chi Gong* can exterminate germs and have manufactured several types of instruments. These imitate the external *Chi* which is emitted by *Chi Gong* masters. The Chinese government permitted research on these abilities because they are considered to be scientific. A few Westerners have visited China to investigate these and some American doctors are learning to practice *Chi Gong* and *T'ai Chi*.

Inner Chi for Energy—Rejuvenation and Longevity—A T'ai Chi Sourcebook presents the idea of doing a gentle regime that can be done in your home or on your patio. The combination of *T'ai Chi* movements and the Microcosmic Meditation is relaxing and healing. They create energy from within the body and are beneficial for longevity and rejuvenation without being tiring.

I invite the reader to go on the computer and Google *T'ai Chi*, *T'ai Chi Chih*, *T'ai Chi Ruler*, *Swimming Dragon*, *Chi Kungs*, etc. Some short videos on You-Tube will be presented. You can check these out and get a feel for some of these movements and see them demonstrated. Select a form you like. Then you can find a teacher in your area as it is always recommended that you start with a class and teacher.

I recommend you also Google *U.S. News and World Report Benefits of T'ai Chi and Chi Gong.* Numerous articles will come up indicating far-reaching research that has been done on the many benefits derived from doing the gentle movements. Participants have benefited from helping heart disease, fibromyalgia, arthritis, Parkinson's, stress, post-traumatic stress disorder, joint health, emotions and balance problems. See the research section at the end of this book.

The practice of these calming and tranquil movements, I hope will be an experience that will send you on a journey into well-being.

When learned correctly and performed regularly, *T'ai Chi* can be a positive part of an overall approach to improving your health.

According to the Mayo Clinic the benefits of *T'ai Chi* include:
- Decreased stress and anxiety
- Increased aerobic capacity
- Increased energy and stamina
- Increased flexibility, balance and agility
- Increased muscle strength and definition

Some evidence indicates that *T'ai Chi* also may help:
- Enhance quality of sleep
- Enhance the immune system
- Lower cholesterol levels and blood pressure
- Improve joint pain
- Improve symptoms of congestive heart failure
- Improve overall well-being in older adults
- Reduce risk of falls in older adults

The ancient man of Tao was subtle, yielding, and childlike. His profound comprehension of the Tao eludes us. Because it is beyond definition, we must recognize it through metaphors:

> *Hesitant and alert, as if crossing a winter stream.*
> *Watchful and aware, as if awaiting unexpected*
> *   encounter from all sides.*
> *Quiet and polite, as if a guest.*
> *Dispersing and subdued, like ice melting away.*
> *Simple and unpretentious, like the 'uncarved block.'*
> *Open and receiving, like the broad valley facing up.*
> *All embracing and unassuming, like muddy water.*

How is it possible to absorb all impurities and remain untainted? By quiescence, just as cloudy water clears when it becomes still.

How can one maintain this quietude and peace? By allowing movement, like the ripples in the settling water.

He who preserves the secret of the Tao lives without exceeding his own needs, content with what he has and what he is.

— *Embrace Tiger, Return to Mountain* by
Al Chuang-liang Huang[1]

A.

T'ai Chi and Qigong
Are Close Relatives

太极

T'ai Chi and Qigong are close relatives and are two forms of meditative movement that have been practiced for thousands of years in China and Tibet for rejuvenation and longevity. For health improvement, they are nearly identical in practical application. In Traditional Chinese Medicine (TCM), they share much in common: posture and movement, breath focus and mind focus (meditative, and mindful). Because of the similarity of T'ai Chi and Qigong, much research now investigates the benefits of both forms together.

T'ai Chi

T'ai Chi translates into "Grand Ultimate." It represents a philosophy that describes the natural world or universe. It was originally developed as a martial art like T'ai Chi Chuan and as a form of meditative movement. Practicing T'ai Chi as meditative movement elicits an internal balance for healing, alleviation of stress, longevity, and personal tranquility. T'ai Chi has become one of the best known movements for refining Qi.

The difference between T'ai Chi and Qigong is that T'ai Chi is performed as a complicated and lengthy (108) series of movements known as T'ai Chi Chuan. Qigong is simpler and easier to learn with more repetitive movements. The practice of the more well-known

T'ai Chi Chuan often will have *Qigong* movements as a warm-up. The basic principles of both forms are body focus, breath focus and mind focus.

In the research on benefits of doing *T'ai Chi*, it is usually not referring to the long form of *T'ai Chi Chuan* but to a modified *T'ai Chi* like *T'ai Chi Easy, T'ai Chi Chih* or short forms with fewer movements. Experts have agreed that it is appropriate to simplify *T'ai Chi* so that people who need movements for physical activity and stress reduction can learn them in a shorter time than the six months to a year or more that it takes to learn the longer 108 movement form of *T'ai Chi Chuan*. The simplified forms of *T'ai Chi* are similar to *Qigong forms* used in health research.

The history of *T'ai Chi* dates back to China in the late 16th century. It is reported that Zhang Sanfeng, a martial artist, created the practice of *T'ai Chi*. According to ancient stories, he had a dream about a snake and a crane in battle and their graceful movements are what inspired his noncombative style of martial arts. Tens of thousands of people in China are still practicing this ancient form every day (and particularly the elderly). In the early 1970s, it was introduced into the United States.

Eastern philosophy believes that *T'ai Chi* unblocks the flow of *Chi*. Health is maintained when *Chi* flows properly and the body, mind and spirit are in balance.

According to *T'ai Chi Overview*, from the University of Maryland Medical School:

> "The three major components of *T'ai Chi* are movement, meditation, and deep breathing.
>
> *Movement*: All the major muscle groups and joints are needed for the slow, gentle movements in *T'ai Chi*. *T'ai Chi* improves balance, agility, strength, flexibility, stamina, muscle tone, and coordination. This low

impact, weight-bearing exercise strengthens bones and can slow bone loss, thus preventing the development of osteoporosis.

Meditation: Research shows that meditation soothes the mind, enhances concentration, reduces anxiety, and lowers blood pressure and heart rate.

Deep breathing: Exhaling stale air and toxins from the lungs while inhaling a plenitude of fresh air increases lung capacity, stretches the muscles involved in breathing and releases tension. It also enhances blood circulation to the brain, which boosts mental alertness. At the same time, the practice supplies the entire body with fresh oxygen and nutrients."

Qigong

Qigong is more ancient than *T'ai Chi*. The original discipline incorporates diverse practices designed to cultivate the enhancement of the life essence that the Chinese call *Qi* or *Chi*. Both *T'ai Chi* and *Qigong* sessions cover a wide range of physical movements that are slow, meditative, and flowing dance-like motions. They both include sitting or standing meditation postures. Both include the regulation of both breath and mind with the body.

Qigong translated from Chinese means to cultivate or enhance the energetic essence of the human being. It is considered to be the modern version of the most ancient healing and medical practices in Asia. Many areas of *Qigong* have a health and medical focus being refined for over 5,000 years.

Doing the *Qigong* movements aids the participants to cultivate *Qi*. *Qi* is the foundation of Traditional Chinese Medicine in acupuncture, herbal medicine and physical therapy. The *Qigong* movements are a series of practices which include body posture, breath, and meditation.

There is external *Qigong* where a medical doctor with *Qigong* will diagnose patients and use *Qi* for healing. The medical doctor may have studied *Qigong* for over five years to develop his energy for healing others. Internal *Qigong* is a personal practice and both affect the balance and flow of energy.

In different regions of China, thousands of forms of *Qigong* practice have been developed during various historic periods. Some forms were for general health purposes, some for Traditional Chinese Medicine (TCM) diagnostic purposes, some for spiritual rituals, and some to gain greater martial arts skill. In the health research, referral is made to simple movements which can be repeated and often flowing with a focused state of relaxed awareness and various breathing techniques.

A key underlying philosophy of the practice is that any form of Qigong has an effect on the cultivation of balance and harmony of Qi, positively influencing the human energy complex (Qi channels/pathways) that functions as a holistic, coherent, and mutually interactive system.

— from *A Comprehensive Review of Health Benefits of Qigong and T'ai Chi* by Roger Jahnke, OMD and Linda Larkey Ph.D., July 21, 2009

B.

What Do *T'ai Chi* and *Qigong* Encompass?

太极

What are the reasons in ancient China and Tibet that the monks daily practiced *T'ai Chi* and *Gigong* movements?

For rejuvenation and longevity.

What is *Qi* or *Chi*?

They are the same way of saying life force energy.

How does *Chi* affect me?

Chi is in all living things. It is life force energy. By doing *T'ai Chi* or *Qigong*, one develops a good strong *Chi*.

What are *Yin* and *Yang*?

Yin and *Yang* are used to describe total universal energy. *Yin* (negative) and *Yang* (positive) charges (female and male) make up the universe. When doing *T'ai Chi* or *Chi Gong*, one balances their energy with *Yin* and *Yang* movements.

What can *Yin* and *Yang* energy be used for?

Yang energy is used in martial arts for self defense. It is expansive and hot and can be used for heating up the body. Too much *Yang* energy becoming very hot can damage organs.

Yin energy is receptive and attractive as a cool energy. It can be used for cooling the body down and for attracting what one wants. One becomes negative if one builds only *Yin* energy and can make one become a victim.

We need both active and receptive energies—both *Yin* and *Yang* movements—for our energies to become balanced The key is balance for power and abilities, happiness, health and a good life force energy.

What is *Chi* breathing?

When you have built your energy, the breath can be used in projecting and amplifying the *Chi*. With the breath, you can direct the energy flow in and out, combining the mind and breath. Then the breath is not used and the mind projects the energy. The breath and the mind work together—where the mind goes, the energy flows.

What is real Yoga or *Qigong* all about?

They are complete sciences of self-transformation with histories going back thousands of years. They are real mind, body spirit sciences that lead to the experience of 'yoga' which means 'union' with the Absolute, the Divine, the Universe. The first step is to connect and feel the *Chi* that is within us and all around us. We must learn to physically experience this energy through practicing real *Qigong* and/or Yoga.

What should I look for in a *T'ai Chi* or *Qigong* teacher?

Can you feel the teacher's *Chi*? Is the teacher emotionally and energetically balanced? Is the teacher non-judgmental?

What is the *Dantian (Dan tien)*?

The *dantian* is translated as 'elixir field' or 'energy center.' *Dantians* are focal points for meditative techniques such as *Qigong* or *T'ai Chi* in Traditional Chinese Medicine. A *dantian* is a center of *Qi* or life-force energy. The lower *dantian* is important as the focal point of breathing techniques and as the center of balance and gravity.

Instruction is often given to remind students to center the mind in the navel or lower *dantian* in order to aid control of thoughts and emotions.

What are the three major *dantians?*

Lower dantian: below the navel three finger widths and two finger widths behind the navel.

Middle dantian: at heart level associated with storing life energy, with respiration and health of internal organs (in particular the thymus gland).

Upper dantian: at forehead between eyebrows (third eye) associated with energy of consciousness and spirit (and with the pineal gland).

What is the importance of the lower *dantian?*

When using the term *dantian*, it is used usually for the lower *dantian*. This is likened to the foundation of rooted standing breath and body awareness in *Gigong*. The term is used in comparison with *hara* in Japan. It is considered the center of gravity of the human body in Chinese, Korean, and Japanese traditions and as the seat of one's internal energy (*Qi*). In the yoga concept, the lower *dantian* corresponds to be the seat of *prana* that radiates outwards to the entire body.

How long is a *T'ai Chi* class?

Group classes usually last an hour. First there is a warm-up phase and then the teacher instructs a series of 20 to 100 *T'ai Chi* movements. The instructor suggests that the students focus on the lower *dantian* and do the movements in a slow and meditative manner focusing on deep breathing. There is often a relaxation or meditation at the end of the class.

What conditions respond well to *T'ai Chi*?

T'ai Chi improves overall fitness, coordination, and agility. People who practice *T'ai Chi* on a regular basis tend to have good posture, flexibility, and range of motion, are more mentally alert, and sleep more soundly at night. (See chapter titled: *T'ai Chi Overview of Benefits*.)

Is *T'ai Chi* safe for most people?

Yes, it is usually safe for everyone and can be modified for many health problems. Many have improved balance and physical performance after six months. It is always wise to talk to your doctor and instructor about health problems.

Experts agree:
"If you want to be healthy and live to 100, do *Qigong*."
— Dr. Mehmet Oz

HISTORICAL BACKGROUND AND PHILOSOPHY

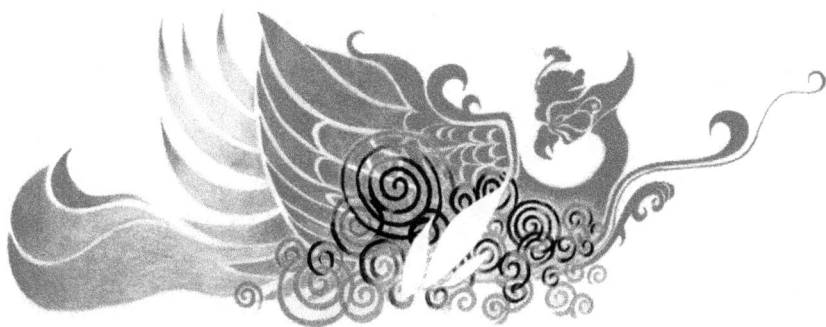

C.

Movements to Generate Energy for Health and Healing

T'ai Chi movements are profound and gentle and encompass the beautifully fluid internal exercises well known to Westerners. It is an exercise program that is part of Traditional Chinese Medicine. *T'ai Chi* is derived from martial arts and includes slow, deliberate movements, meditation, and deep breathing. However, breathing should be effortless.

By doing them, you feel a surge of vital force in the body, a tingling in the fingers and a feeling of power. *T'ai Chi* has the special quality of the interaction of softness and energetic movements that is in accord with the theory of the mutual complement of *Yin* and *Yang*. *T'ai Chi* is known as the *internal school*, emphasizing soft, graceful, fluid movements that are similar to dancing. In contrast, the *external school* movements known as martial arts are sometimes hard and vigorous, involving much leaping, kicking and somersaulting.

According to legend, *T'ai Chi* was founded by Taoist Master Chang San-feng (or Sanfeng). He was known by many names. It is reported he lived to be 200 years old (1247–1447). By the 1870s, the Yang family, *Tai Chi Chuan* teachers, were claiming that Chang San-Feng was the originator of *Tai Chu Chuan*. In any event, he was probably a highly respected Taoist master of an internal style of martial arts.

T'ai Chi has been practiced in China for over 3,000 years. It can be described as a moving meditation. In China, some ten million people practice some form of *T'ai Chi* daily. It is usually practiced outdoors at dawn. Classes begin with a few minutes of standing meditation to calm the mind and to gather energy. The two popular versions of *T'ai Chi Chuan* have 18 and 37 movements. It takes some time to learn the forms which are done in a relaxed manner and are connected with circular movements, one flowing into the next.

The internal movements are gentle forms of shadowboxing and swordplay, but with the emphasis on fluidity. They coordinate breathing with movements to prevent illness, stressing relaxation, tranquility and naturalness, thereby promoting strength and grace.

For centuries, the Chinese have had a great understanding of the relationship between mind and body. As a health exercise, the internal exercises like *T'ai Chi* are suitable for both men and women, old and young, weak and strong, due to the softness, slowness, coherence and harmony of the movements. It is a form that engages the mind and spirit in patterns of great beauty.

Traditionally, the ultimate purpose of practicing these exercises was to achieve longevity and eternal youth. For example, a master of *T'ai Chi Chuan* in his 80s can fight off a much younger man. Mental and physical responses remain strong into the 80s and 90s.

Consistent practice will improve one's health because the movements stimulate the circulatory, lymphatic and immune systems as well as the central nervous system. *T'ai Chi* circulates energy (*Chi*) through the meridians. The strength of the bones and muscles and the functions of the metabolic, respiratory and cardiovascular systems are greatly improved.

The key to the effectiveness of the movements is in the slowness, which actually increases the energy in the body. Inner stillness also aids in developing awareness. It relaxes the nerves and releases anxiety and tension. *T'ai Chi* promotes harmony of the mind and body.

The movements improve physiological functions, enabling its students to become fit and maintain a normal life as they get older. The configuration of *T'ai Chi* is the circular combination of *Yin* and *Yang* in a flow that is always evolving, separating in movement and combining in stillness. They use mind and not force. In Taoism, the circle is called *Wu Chi*, the origin of the universe, the Mother of *Yin* and *Yang*.

By using abdominal breathing, one increases one's vital capacity by lowering the diaphragm and increasing and adjusting the oxygen supply needed in the body. The muscles of the abdomen are thereby strengthened, and peristaltic movement is stimulated in the intestines. A moderate amount of internal movement may increase the oxygen-loading capacity of the heart muscle and help rehabilitate it after coronary illness.

The five essential qualities of *T'ai Chi* are:

Slowness	To develop awareness
Lightness	To make movements flow
Balance	To prevent body strain
Calmness	To maintain continuity
Clarity	To focus the mind

The benefits from practicing *T'ai Chi* are both physical and mental. Done regularly, *T'ai Chi* improves muscle tone, flexibility, balance, and coordination. Older people have discovered that it increases their energy and agility, sharpens their reflexes and they have an overall feeling of well-being. Some have used it for healing and as an addition to other programs for chronic conditions of arthritis, fibromyalgia or heart disease. Research has discovered that *T'ai Chi* often holds a person's interest longer than other types of exercise and it is safe for people of all ages and fitness abilities.

T'ai Chi and *Gigong* movements have been used for centuries in China and Tibet for rejuvenation, longevity, stress relief, and healing. The West is just learning about these gentle internal movements that greatly benefit one's physical and mental health.

D.

Yin and *Yang*

太极

Yin and *Yang* are two forms of how *Chi* energy manifests. Everything in nature involves the flow and balance of *Yin* and *Yang* as complementary forms of energy. The health of the organs depends upon the flow of *Chi* and upon the proper balance of *Yin* and *Yang* within each organ and meridian system. Illness occurs when the flow of *Chi* along a meridian is obstructed or when the balance of *Yin* and *Yang* within an organ is upset. *Ch'i kung* exercises help to maintain the flow of vital energy and to maintain proper *Yin/Yang* balance within the organs.

The symbol represents the "Tao" or *T'ai Chi* which is the Supreme Ultimate. The white is the *Yang* force, which is heat, expansion, the creative, male, positive. The black is the *Yin* force, which is cold, contractive, receptive, female, negative. (See page 27.)

YANG	*T'AI-CHI*	*YIN*
Heaven	Man	Earth
Parent	Adult	Child
Sun	Day / Night	Moon
Body	Spirit	Mind
Physical	Feelings	Mental
Hard	Resilient	Soft
Expand	Pulsation	Contract
Right Brain/Body	Whole Brain/Body	Left Brain/Body
Back Body	Whole Body	Front Body

T'ai Chi Symbol (Taijitu)

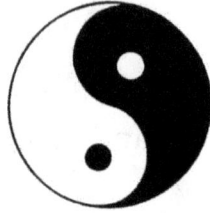

The *T'ai Chi* symbol, the Taijitu, is known as the *Yin/Yang* symbol. In the book *Written in Stone*[4], the Triptych pattern is the chief architectural symbol of the doctrine of "harmony-through-the-balance-of-opposites" which is an ancient occult/alchemical philosophy shared worldwide. The Taijitu and the Triptych both emphasize the number three.

In China, this doctrine is expressed in the age-old Chinese religious tradition of Taoism, whose main goal is "harmony-through-the-balance-of-opposites."

> *The Chinese trinity, being the duality of yang and yin organized into a higher unity under the harmonious influence of Chi, is regarded as the source of all existence and its symbol ... possesses a deep religious significance for the Chinese heart.*
>
> — Lao Tzu

When first looking at the Taijitu, it does not look like a tripartite symbol, but it does represent a trinity. The white half *Yang*, symbolizes the universal active, aggressive, "male" forces. The black half *Yin*, is the universe's passive, receptive or "female" forces.

The circle is the third power reconciling the *Yin/Yang* opposites. The circle is a return to their unity. In Chinese thought, this is called the "Tao", the all-encompassing circle. The circle being a shape that stands for eternity with no beginning and no end.

28

What is the meaning of the entire T'ai-Chi diagram? The T'ai-Chi diagram illustrates how two opposites can be harmonized into a whole interrelated unit. Like other principles of T'ai-Chi, this one can apply to natural as well as human relationships.

For example, positive and negative polarities in electricity can be seen in terms of Yin and Yang harmony. Neither a positive electric charge nor a negative one can separately produce light or heat. These opposites need each other to become electricity, just as both Yin and Yang are necessary to form a T'ai-Chi unity.

　　　　— The Tao of T'ai-Chi Chuan, *Way to Rejuvenation* by Jou, Tsung Hwa[2]

Yin/Yang Theory in Traditional Chinese Medicine

According to Denise Aughtman, Doctor of Oriental Medicine, San Miguel de Allende, Guanajuato, Mexico:

The theory of harmony between Yin Qi and Yang Qi is the essence of Chinese Medicine, and is the foundational training of doctors of Chinese Medicine. This foundation of Chinese Medicine is over 3,000 years old.

The relationship of Yin and Yang (literal translation: shadow and light) is used to describe how opposite, or contrary, elemental forces are related, interconnected, and interdependent in the natural world. This elemental theory is the foundation of Traditional Chinese Medicine.

Many natural dualities—dark and light, feminine and masculine, low and high, cold and hot, water and fire—are some of the physical manifestations of the relationship between Yin and Yang.

Yin and Yang are not separate forces, but inter-related and complementary, and create a synergistic whole that is greater than the individual Yin or Yang. This principle generates a beautiful and dynamic system where every living thing is made up of the inter-related aspects of Yin and Yang, which are mutually interdependent—shadow cannot exist without light, masculine cannot exist without feminine, etc.

Traditional Chinese Medicine assesses and treats imbalances within the relationship of Yin and Yang by differentiating patient symptoms according to five inter-related elements. Once imbalances of these elements are assessed, Acupuncture and Chinese Herbal Medicine specifically treat the disharmony of Yin Qi and Yang Qi, resulting in the five-element harmony of the patient. This is the foundational theory of Traditional Chinese Medicine.

E.

Chi (Energy)

太极

Chi is associated with breath and energy and is the foundation of Chinese philosophy. *T'ai Chi* Master Wen-Shan Huang has stated that it has never been scientifically analyzed. In ancient Chinese classics there are more than sixty terms that stand for *Chi*.

> "In Lao Tzu's cosmogeny, it seems that the Tao begot One, and that One is Chi, which, in turn, begot the Two—YIN and YANG—which then led to Heaven, Earth, and Man. Hence, Lao Tzu, in his *Tao Teh Ching*, said:
>
> > *The TAO begot One,*
> > *One begot Two,*
> > *Two begot Three,*
> > *And Three begot ten thousand things.*
> > *The ten thousand things carry YIN and embrace*
> >   *YANG;*
> > *They achieve harmony by combining these forces.*
>
> Based on this passage, it is evident that TAO is Absolute and begot the two *Chis* of YIN and YANG. With the interaction of these two forces, there appeared a state of harmony in which everything emerged. All things carry YIN in the back and

embrace YANG in the front. The blending together of the two *Chi's* of YIN and YANG achieve a new harmony. Thus we see that, quite early, the Chinese sages endeavored to establish some kind of cosmology based upon the concepts of TAO, *Chi*, and YIN-YANG.

Chi, then, to the *Wu Chi* Taoist, is not some mysterious force that exists somewhere in another world and has to be summoned by rituals or magic. It is a living, viable force that surrounds and permeates all things.

When one has finally attained the highest stage of maturity in the training of *T'ai Chi Chu'an*, one has gone beyond the prolonging of life and warding off of disease. Then so-called 'supernatural power,' or spiritual strength, may be realized."[3]

When you do the gentle movements of *T'ai Chi,* your hands begin to feel a vibration after only a few of the forms. After the session, you have more energy than before. The *Chi* is also circulated through the body for health and healing with the Microcosmic Orbit Meditation.

BREATH—*To Gather the Ch'i*

*If the ch'i is dispersed, then it is not stored (accumulated)
and is easy to scatter. Let the ch'i penetrate the spine and the
inhalation and exhalation be smooth and unimpeded
throughout the entire body. The inhalation closes and
gathers, the exhalation opens and discharges. Because the
inhalation can naturally raise and also uproot the opponent,
the exhalation can naturally sink down and also discharge
him. This is by means of the i (mind), not the li (strength)
mobilizing the ch'i (breath).*

> — *The Essence of T'ai Chi Ch'uan, The
> Literary Tradition*[5]

F.

Chinese Medicine—
Chi and Meridians

太极

One of the well-known forms of *Chi Kungs* is "The Swimming Dragon." T.K. Shih in his book, *The Swimming Dragon,* comments that *Chi Kung* belongs to a large family of Chinese exercises designed to cultivate, circulate and store vital energy, promote longevity, and improve health. *Chi* means vital energy, that which animates both mind and body. *Kung* means exercise as well as time spent in performing the exercises. *Chi* is often spelled *Qi* or, in its Japanese form, *ki.*[6]

The Swimming Dragon is a lovely *Chi Kung* and can be a daily practice. Google it and also look it up on YouTube. It takes a little longer to learn than some of the other forms.

Ch'i Kung and Chinese Medicine

According to T.K. Shih the *Ch'i Kung* practices are based on ancient principles of Chinese medicine. It is a sophisticated system for maintaining good health, preventing and curing disease and also increasing general vitality and well-being. The author has been a medical doctor for over fifty years and believes the most effective way of gaining and maintaining health and vitality is by cultivating *Chi* energy through the practice of *Ch'i Kung*.

An excerpt from *The Swimming Dragon*[6]:

Chinese medicine is based on the ideas that a living being is an energy system, and that all life is based on *chi*. There are many different forms of energy in the universe and many special forms of *chi* that flow through our body. These different kinds of energy are connected to our bodily organs and flow in a system of channels called meridians and collaterals. The system of the twelve meridians and eight collaterals and the differentiation of *chi* energy into *Yin* and *Yang* phases form the basis of Chinese medicine and all *Ch'i-Kung* or energy exercises. Each meridian is associated with one of the main body organs. In Chinese medicine, the name of each organ refers not only to the physical organ given by the name of heart, lung, liver, large intestine, etc., but to the whole system of energy and energy flow that derives from that organ. Each organ has its characteristic energy of *ch'i* and it is this energy that flows through the meridians.

The meridians pass through the arms, legs, body and trunk and connect with their associated organs. Six meridians flow through the arms and six through the legs. Along the meridians are the acupuncture points. These are precise locations that can be used to regulate the functioning of the organ/meridian systems. The meridians can be stimulated or sedated by massaging the acupuncture points, by the application of heat or needles to these points, and most importantly, through *ch'i-kung* practices.

Vitality depends not only upon the flow and balance of *chi* but its abundance as well. *Ch'i-kung* practice is concerned with increasing the quantity of *chi* energy and storing it in the channels called collaterals and in the three storage vessels known as *tan tiens*: upper *tan t'ien* (third eye), middle *tan t'ien* (solar plexus), and lower *tan t'ien* (approximately 2" below navel).

Meridians

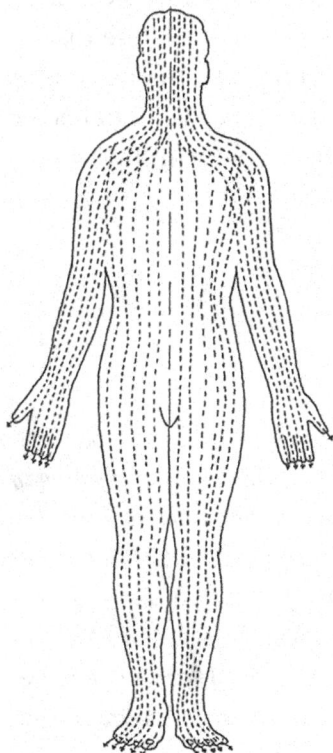

The collaterals are eight channels (or extraordinary meridians) that store energy. The three *tan t'iens* are areas that are connected with energy. The *tan t'iens* are located in the centers of the head, chest and abdomen. As you do the *Ch'i Kung* movements, the collaterals and *tan t'iens* become full. This energy then becomes available to go to the meridians/organ systems. *Chi* takes three different forms: It is called *ching* in the lower *tan t'ien*, *Chi* when in the middle *tan t'ien*, and *shen* when in the upper *tan t'ien*. *Ching* is a strong form of energy associated with sexual energy and capable of manifesting externally as sperm and sexual fluids.

37

Chi proper does not manifest in any external material form, but is experienced as it circulates through the body. *Shen,* like *Chi,* cannot be perceived externally, but is experienced subjectively as a feeling of clarity and alertness. These three forms of energy are capable of being transformed into one another: *Ching* becomes *Chi* and *Chi* becomes *shen.* But *shen* also can become *Chi,* and *Chi,* once generated and in circulation, can be stored in the lower *tan t'ien* as *ching.*

The principle of Yin and Yang is the basis of the entire Universe. It is the principle of everything in creation. It brings about the transformation to parenthood; it is the root and source of Life and Death. Heaven was created by an accumulation of Yang; the Earth was created by an accumulation of Yin. The ways of Yin and Yang are to the left and to the right. Water and fire are the symbols of Yin and Yang, and are the source of power of everything in Creation.

Yang ascends to Heaven; Yin descends to Earth. Hence, the Universe (Heaven and Earth) represents motion and rest, controlled by the wisdom of nature. Nature grants the power to beget and to grow, to harvest and to store, to finish and to begin anew.

— *Yin and Yang* by Huang Ti Nei Ching Su Wen[3]

The Eight Branches of Oriental Medicine

It is interesting to see where *Gi Gong* and *T'ai Chi* fit into the overall structure of Oriental Medicine.

From Denise Aughtman, Doctor of Oriental Medicine, San Miguel de Allende, Guanajuato, Mexico:

I offer thanks to the Taoist practitioners of old for their efforts, empiricism and devotion to discover an effective lifestyle to generate vitality and preserve longevity. Then, as now, human culture desired vibrant health and longevity. The Taoists of that time brought this practice to the world along with the Tao, or the balanced One. They shared the Eight Branches of Oriental Medicine rather than just managing symptoms. It includes the peace and harmony of body, emotion, mind, spirit—all aspects of being human.

The eight branches of Oriental medicine are:
1. Meditation
2. Preventative medicine for vitality
3. Acupuncture and moxibustion
4. Herbal medicine and tonics
5. Diagnosis using the Five Elements
6. Feng Shui
7. Qi Gong and T'ai Chi
8. Therapeutic massage

The metaphor of Eight Branches refers to Root Medicine. If the roots of the tree are healthy, the branches will be healthy and bear fruit. Over three thousand years, the Eight Branches of Oriental Medicine have proven to generate balanced vitality of health and create longevity.

G.

T'ai Chi and
Chi Kung Principles

太极

As *T'ai Chi* and *Chi Kung* have been done for many years for rejuvenation and longevity, certain principles are important to learn. To become acquainted with a few of the estimated 70,000 different *Chi Kungs*, you can go on YouTube or Google *T'ai Chi* or *Chi Kung*.

One site is *Movement Arts* by Dan Kleiman which lists "5 YouTube *Qigong* Videos You Can Actually Learn From," November 28, 2011.

It was interesting for me to compare some of the movements with ones I had learned in *T'ai Chi Chih*:

"Simple Circling Hands" is similar to "Bass Drum."

"Transitioning into More Movement" is similar to "Daughter on the Mountain Top." (The body is lower and the hands cross.)

"Rolling the Ball" is similar to "Passing Clouds." (The hands are different.)

• • •

Dr. Paul Lam at the *T'ai Chi for Health Institute* has listed some guiding principles.

He states that the first thing that sets *T'ai Chi* apart from other martial arts is that it is an *internal art*. *T'ai Chi* involves the mind, the inside body and the inner power, the *Qi*. We have to focus on our movements and this helps us to integrate our mind and body, to constantly use our minds to analyze the movement. That helps us to practice intelligently.

The next principle is *Integration* which means whenever you move, your mind and body is integrated. Are the hand, trunk, and foot all fully coordinated at a given point of time? One part of the body moves and the rest follow.

> "The very core of T'ai Chi is Balance, balance of
> movements, of yin and yang and of internal and
> external. Too soft or too harsh are both not well
> balanced; a movement that stretches so far that you
> nearly fall is not good T'ai Chi … Another example is
> too much emphasis on relaxation. This is very
> important but if you are so soft and so relaxed like
> a jelly, then there is no strength. That to me is
> imbalance with only too much yin and not
> enough yang."

Dr. Lam defines:

Dantian: The *Dantian* is in the center of the body and is the center of *Qi*. It is two to three finger-breadths below the belly button and two inches inwards. An essential part of *T'ai Chi* is to practice the awareness of the *dantian* and sinking *Qi* to the *Dantian*.

Practice: One of the "absolute always stay true" principles is practice. If you do not practice, you will not understand the inner meaning of *T'ai Chi* and not benefit completely from it.

Conclusion: Most people are learning *T'ai Chi* for health. One needs to be strong inside and outside and also have more clarity in the mind. With the combination of stronger *Qi* and better balance of body and mind, this works both for health and martial arts. Decide what your goal is and you will direct your efforts and your learning toward what is most effective for you.

• • •

On YouTube, also view the *T'ai Chi Chih* video by Justin Stone—*T'ai Chi Chih Principles*:

This is the sequence that I first learned and it is a great way to start your exploration and perhaps your continuing practice of *T'ai Chi*. Justin Stone developed the 20 movements of *T'ai Chi Chih* in 1974 based on ancient forms and presents the principles in this video.

Justin states that *T'ai Chi Chih* is not an exercise. Do it loosely and without effort. Do it softly. Softness is very important and the more you practice this, the more benefits you will get from it. The *Chi*, the energy, that is circulating in the body, will be blocked if there is tension. The *Chi* flows softly and there are benefits from it.

When you start your movements, the fingers are apart and you start to move. Watch the waist and the wrists, and the torso is kept absolutely still, and your head suspended from the ceiling. Feel you are swimming through very heavy air. Do it in a very leisurely fashion, do not rush, the waist pivots and the arms move with no effort.

The hips do swivel when you do the movement in "Carry the Ball." The hips do the work, not the arms. The arms and the body move together.

The shifting of the weight is important. Going forward in the *T'ai Chi* Step, the front leg is substantial (it stiffens) and the back leg is insubstantial.

Learn three or four movements to begin and practice them daily. Then learn three or four more. Then soon you will have twenty movements and can practice them every day.

There are factors that you can tell if you are making progress. The first is that your fingers may start to flutter (the energy is flowing through you). The second sign comes when you are doing the movements after some time and you realize that the movements are doing themselves. *T'ai Chi Chih* is doing *T'ai Chi Chih*! The third confirming sign may take a few years. You will be able to do the movements mentally.

The most important principle is to practice every day. Practice when you feel like it and practice when you don't feel like it! The practice of *T'ai Chi Chih* promotes feelings of well-being, relaxation, inner peace and serenity.

I have chosen to be happy,
because it is good for my health.
— Voltaire

H.

The Importance of the
Tan Tien (Dantian)

太极

Tan tien, dantian, dan t'ian, dan tien is translated as "elixir field" or energy center. These areas are important focal points for exercise and meditative techniques in *Gigong, T'ai Chi, T'ai Chi Chuan* and Traditional Chinese Medicine. A *tan tien* is considered to be a center of *Qi* or *Chi*. The lower *dantian* is important as central points in breathing techniques and as the center of balance and gravity.

Traditional *T'ai Chi* and *Gigong* masters (Taoist and Buddhist) would instruct students to center the mind in the navel or lower *dantian*. They believed it aided in control of thoughts and emotions. *Dantians* are considered major storage areas of *Chi*.

The three major *dantians*:

Lower dantian below the navel about three finger widths below and two finger widths behind the navel.

Middle dantian at the level of the heart (associated with storing life energy and with respiration and health of the internal organs and with the thymus gland).

Upper dantian at the forehead between the eyebrows or third eye (associated with energy of consciousness and spirit *shen* and with the pineal gland).

The *dantian*, your power center, is like an energetic heart. It has the same function for the energy as your heart has for the blood circulation. When you feel your *dantian* and relax your body, you are ready for the right posture which influences the flow of *Chi* in your body. You are ready to feel energy when you combine relaxation, *dantian* and the right posture. Proper breathing is also a key for relaxation and well-being.

You can use your *dantian* to make the *Chi* flow in the body and to protect yourself. When you are centered, you feel rooted and have a central axis of the body. You can imagine a heavy ball in your belly. If you are sensitive, you can feel your center. Direct your attention to the *dantian* in order to feel it. When you are doing *T'ai Chi* or *Chi Gong* movements, it is important to connect to the *dantian*. You do this with regular practice. It is the basic and main tool to all *Chi* techniques. It is the place where *Chi* is purified before sending it to flow in the body. It is the only place where it is safe to gather energy. The *Chi* needs to flow freely. If the *Chi* flows too fast, you can feel dizzy. You can slow the flow by contracting your center.

When you become completely relaxed, put your *attention* and *intention* on your *dantian*. A basic technique and exercise for all inner techniques of *Chi* is to practice pushing it forward in the lower belly with the inhale and bringing it back to the center with the exhale. Feel it in the center and start breathing from the *dantian* and fill your entire body with each inhale and then take everything back to center with the exhale. If you have it contracted all day, you will be in the right posture. It is the center of control and therefore regulates the *Chi* (life energy).

It is very important to become conscious of the *dantian*. The body organizes itself around it when you are connected and centered. Being the gravity center, it connects you to all gravity centers in the universe. The body becomes strong and efficient with less effort, making you powerful, calm and rooted. It brings you to the *here and now.*

Relax and take your time to combine all these elements. You can start with five minutes a day, then ten minutes and after a few months can be practicing *T'ai Chi* or *Gi Gong* for thirty minutes a day.

Before learning the specific movements, the student is well-advised to observe and to cultivate each of the following principles of the T'ai Chi Chi Kung:

1. Be natural, quiet and relaxed.

2. Combine the will and the Chi.

3. Establish solidity in the lower body and legs.

4. Move slowly and cultivate stability.

5. Practice diligently and regularly.

6. Observe moderation in the extent of movement.

— Jou, Tsung Hwa., *The Tao of T'ai-Chi Chuan, Way to Rejuvenation*[2]

I.

Literary References
to *T'ai Chi Chuan*[5]

太极

"In motion all parts of the body must be
light, nimble and strung together.

• • •

Walk like a cat.

• • •

Be still as a mountain
move like a great river.

• • •

The motion should be rooted in the feet,
released through the legs,
controlled by the waist,
and manifested through the fingers.
The feet, legs and waist
must act together simultaneously
so that while stepping forward or back
the timing and position are correct.
If the timing and position are not correct,
the body becomes disordered,
and the defect must be sought
in the legs and waist.

• • •

Ch'ang Ch'uan (*T'ai Chi Ch'uan*)
is like a great river rolling on unceasingly.

• • •

Remember, when moving,
there is no place that doesn't move.
When still,
there is no place that isn't still.
First seek extension,
then contraction;
then it can be fine and subtle.
It is said 'if others don't move,
I don't move.
If others move slightly,
I move first'.

• • •

The form is like that
of a falcon about to seize a rabbit,
and the *shen* (spirit) is like that
of a cat about to catch a rat.

• • •

Study the function of each posture
carefully and with deliberation;
to achieve the goal is very easy.
Pay attention to the waist at all times;
completely relax the abdomen
and the *ch'i* (breath) rise up.
When the coccyx is straight,
the *shen* (spirit) goes through to the headtop.
To make the whole body light and agile,
suspend the headtop."

J.

Taoism

Da Liu states in his book *T'ai Chi Ch'uan and I Ching* that:

The concept of yin and yang is often associated with the name of Lao-tzu. Actually, it was discovered and used for something like 4,800 years, several thousand years before Lao-tzu and his famous work, the Tao Teh Ching, which enunciated the principles of Taoism. The polarities of yin and yang exist everywhere, in everything and in every time. In the I Ching and Taoist thought, heaven is yang, earth is yin, sun is yang, moon is yin, man is yang, woman is yin, firmness is yang, yielding is yin. In the body, the head is yang and the belly is yin. Since this duality penetrates all of nature, we can, of course, find many examples.

Lao-tzu, although not the inventor of this concept, expounded it magnificently. He lived between 604 and 531 B.C., though legend has it that he lived to be several hundred years old. In his youth, he was supposedly a librarian who kept documents in the time of the Chu Dynasty. But he gave up his job and went to live alone as a hermit in far West China. He is said to have been the Immortal who passed on to Buddha the secret of immortality. Legend also has it that he met Confucius and awed him by his superior wisdom. Whatever the validity of these stories, Lao-tzu expounded the philosophy of the Tao most eloquently.

He who follows the Tao
is one with the Tao.
— Lao Tzu

Being at one with the Tao is eternal,
though the body dies,
the Tao will never pass away.
— Lao Tzu

DOING THE MOVEMENTS

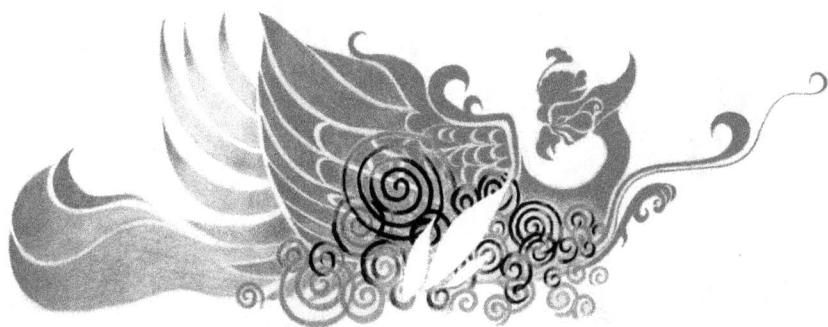

K.

Strengthening Our
Chi Connection

太极

Relaxation is the Core of Chi Kung and T'ai Chi

In doing our *T'ai Chi* movements, we are so happy to feel the *Chi* (the energy) in our fingertips and body. We now learn that *Chi* has quality as well as quantity. The *Chi* picks up outside information that changes its pure inner signal. How can we restore the right signal to the *Chi?*

The body thrives when it receives the pure original signal. Otherwise, wrong signals infect our *Chi* and are broadcast to each cell in our body causing decline and suffering. *Chi* serves as a bridge between mind and body. If you hold angry thoughts in your mind, you can create physical sensations in your gut. According to the ancient Taoists, *Chi* is the only bridge between the mind and body and the outside world.

It is recommended the less thinking the better when doing *T'ai Chi*. It is best to use the pure mind of a baby. The source of truth is the feeling of our life energy. By preferring thinking, we pick up wrong programming. It requires hard work to wake up the ability to trust our original energy. The ancient monks encouraged people to keep their minds calm and reduce interaction with the outside world. They were teaching them to protect their life energy.

Chi flows throughout your body affecting every cell, mood and thought. You can smooth and clean your life energy through *Chi*

Kung—teaching one how to focus, relax and stay calm. How do we restore our life energy? Your life energy was strong, fresh and new when you were a baby! It had the pattern for perfect function. All the thinking and the education has contaminated the original pristine life energy.

Understanding the power of that single cell is important. Losing that power is one of the reasons we age, get ill and die. We still have that original single cell signal deep inside us. The force of life is created in that single cell through the power of flow which splits into two. A third power is created between and around the cells. It grows as the cells continue to multiply. The third force is your *Chi* and holds each part together. It has the ability to communicate to all the cells in your body. This is of great importance to commit to, purify and strengthen your *Chi* through *Chi Kung* and *T'ai Chi*.

In the year 300 A.D. before it acquired the name *T'ai Chi* from Master Chang San Feng in the 13th century, the earliest Taoist temples were using moving meditation. The further forward we go in life, the signal of life energy becomes fainter. To go backward and return to this center, then all wisdom, true power and real transformation is ours. The monks worked to strip away everything in their minds, their lives and energy that wasn't pure.

The old Taoist masters understood the value of the *Chi* connection—to heal the body they must go through the *Chi*. Through ongoing practice of *T'ai Chi* moving meditation and *Chi Kung* exercises, we gradually send a message through our *Chi* to help, restore, rebalance and wake up dormant cells before we reach the disease state. Every step you take to make your lifestyle more natural will help your *Chi* connection.

What is the key element shared by *Chi Kung*, *T'ai Chi* and *Tao Gung*? They all rely on moving meditation. *Chi* is our life energy and that energy is created and supported by the piece of God's energy inside of us. Life energy is alive and living things move.

Of all the ancient wisdom traditions, *Chi Kung, T'ai Chi* and *Tao Gung* are so powerful! They maintain the only systems that preserve the wisdom of moving meditation. Move and meditate. Our *Chi* knows exactly what our bodies need and how to repair them. We need to restore our *Chi* awareness. We use feeling as we move. Through moving meditation, we reconnect to our true life energy feeling. We gradually clean up our energy layer by layer until we get down to that original signal.

Focusing on the lower *tan tien* (lower stomach) is important—part of going backward. Your mother's womb was the cradle of life for you. We return to the *tan tien* to wake up that memory, reminding our energy to return home. Movements are round and follow a natural curve. Encourage *Chi* to flow the natural way—relaxed and gentle. Relaxation is the core of *Chi Kung* and *T'ai Chi*.

We can learn to flow our *Chi* inside our body to where it hurts. Start with hands, arms shoulders and continue in body. Start to expand. Flow the feeling as a pure calm mind. If you want to learn more about your flow of *Chi* and energy in the body see the book, *Restoring Your Life Energy* by Waysun Liao.[7]

L.

Tan Tien
Moving Meditation

太极

This standing meditation can be adapted to sitting or walking or waiting in line. You can use it when you want to bring yourself back to a more centered feeling of harmony. You never do this if you are angry or upset. This will also help you clean your *Chi* (your energy).

Locate the center of each palm and concentrate your attention there for a few minutes. Bring your hands in front of your lower *tan tien*.

Inhale and exhale from that area and feel as if a ball is there. As you inhale, an imaginary ball expands very slightly. As you exhale, it gets smaller. As you exhale, follow the shrinking ball and bring your hands back closer to your *tan tien*. Your hands never touch your stomach—they are always a few inches away.

Concentrate on the center of your palms beaming energy toward your *tan tien*. Feel the imaginary ball in your lower stomach area expand and contract as you inhale and exhale.

M.

T'ai Chi
Movement Preparation

太极

Before doing any movements, remind yourself that these internal forms of exercise emphasize slow movements and tranquility of mind. The underlying principle is that action follows thought. All internal exercises are controlled by such consciousness, so one must therefore be quiet and calm before beginning and then apply one's total concentration. Relaxation is all important. Muscles and joints need to be relaxed so that all rigidity disappears. The torso is kept upright, with arms rounded and knees flexed. Concentrate on the soles of the feet or the lower *tan t'ien*.

Special attention is paid to balance. Lightness and suppleness characterize the movements. They should be done slowly and smoothly, as the motions are in accord with the natural movements of the body. The movements require close coordination of the upper and lower parts of the body. You must be aware of your breathing. These well-coordinated movements involve the whole body.

You will find a natural rhythm with the movements after they have become more automatic. You will be able to follow the *Chi* energies as they move throughout the body, often from specified points above you, from the earth, from surrounding space, from the stars. You may feel them mix in the lower *tan t'ien* and circulate and radiate back out into the environment. With practice you will be able to specifically expand your capacity to receive and radiate love as part of the *Chi* energy. Accumulating power in the body has long been understood as part of these movements. It is less understood that one can combine this with love.

While moving, pay special attention to certain parts of the body. Move your head naturally with your torso; keep your chin in and mouth closed, with your tongue resting gently behind your upper teeth. Breathe through your nose. Your neck should neither be too stiff nor too relaxed. The hands are slightly cupped, with the fingers spread apart. Your chest should be pulled in and your shoulders kept low. Gravity acts through your legs and gives you firm contact with the ground. Knee joints are relaxed throughout and are never locked. You are 'Yinging' and 'Yanging' with the legs.

Remember to move the whole body forward and move the whole body backward; turn the whole body by rotating the pelvis. Do not use strength; use *Chi* and the mind.

N.

T'ai Chi
Practice Tips

太 极

1. Stand quietly a few moments before beginning. Relax the entire body and calm the mind. Allow the weight to rest on your feet.

2. Concentrate your mind in the direction of movement. The mind leads and the body follows in its natural order.

3. Imagine the head suspended by a golden cord from above, keeping the spine long, let the chest remain relaxed and low, the shoulders easy, torso vertical and elbows sunk.

4. When you step, be aware of the space between your two feet. Step lightly and balance like a cat.

5. Movement continues in a slow, even tempo. Movements are circular.

6. Use your waist as an axis and imagine your arms as the spokes of a wheel. To turn the waist is to turn the shoulders; they are connected and one cannot be turned without the other.

7. Drop and relax your shoulders; do not raise and lower them. Elbows are always lower than the hands if the hands are above the waist. Dropping your elbows will help you relax your shoulders.

8. Keep the posture low. Sink your center of gravity to the lower abdomen.

9. Arms must be relaxed and rounded. Keep arms in front of and away from the body, never touching the chest.

10. Breathe easily and naturally through the nose. Focus your attention on each movement.

11. While doing the movements, keep your tongue against the roof of the mouth.

Summary for *T'ai Chi Chih*[8] movements:

Concentrate on soles of feet or lower *tan t'ien*. The Chinese start on left side. Pause three to four seconds between a series of nine movements on both left and right sides; i.e., allowing the *Yin* and *Yang* to come together. Eyelids can be half closed; look diagonally in front to the floor but do not bend the head. *Stay relaxed and imagine you are swimming through very heavy air.* The hands are slightly cupped and the fingers a little apart. For the Chinese, 9 is a positive number, so the movements are performed 9, 18, or 36 times to one's left and then to one's right. End each set with a graceful conclusion, which is a gentle dip at the knees, palms down in front of the lower *tan t'ien*. Center yourself. Stand quietly and bring your attention and energy within. Take a couple of deep breaths.

O.

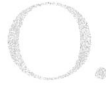

T'ai Chi Warmups
(Commonly included with many *chi kung* movements.)

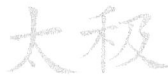

太极

1. **Four gates:** With neck relaxed, turn your head to the right, go back to center, then chin up, back to center, then to the left, back to center, and then chin down, repeat.

2. **Head rolls:** Very slowly roll your head starting at right shoulder, down in front and then to left shoulder. Go slowly from left shoulder to right shoulder.

3. **Shoulder Rolls:** Very slowly and gently roll your shoulders to the front and up to the ears, and then back, and come around making a circle. Do this several times in one direction and then reverse direction.

4. **Arm Circles:** Very slowly make large arm circles starting with your right arm, and go backwards (left leg forward). Do this three times and then reverse direction. Then with the left arm, make three slow circles forward and then back (right leg forward).

5. **Knee Rotations:** Bend over and place your palms on your knees and slowly rotate the knees one direction three or four times and then reverse directions.

6. **Opening Breath:** Place palms together at heart level:

Inhale and separate palms (still facing each other) to shoulder width.

Exhale, turn palms downward and push them toward the earth. Knees sink at same time. Rotate wrists so that palms face upward (fingertips forward).

Inhale and pull palms up to shoulders (fingertips still forward).

Exhale and rotate wrists outwards (palms still upward with fingertips pointing backward) and push upward directly overhead.

Rotate wrists (palms face each other, fingertips point upward).

Inhale and lower extended arms to shoulder level at sides (palms upward).

Exhale and extend arms (palms face each other). Bring palms together one inch apart in front of chest.

Inhale, rotate wrists (palms downward) and pull wrists toward shoulders.

Exhale and push palms toward the earth to return to center position.

Inhale and bring hands back up to shoulders and repeat from start.

P.

T'ai Chi Step
(for *T'ai Chi Chih*)

太极

A basic step used in many of the movements. The motion is slow and smooth, shifting the weight forward and back, thus circulating and balancing the *Chi* in the body. One knee is bent and the other leg relaxed and straight. The spine and head remain aligned as they shift forward and back. The substantial (*Yang*) leg is the leg that supports the body; the other leg is called the insubstantial (*Yin*). The movements always start with the left leg forward, and there is a pronounced heel-and-toe motion so that when the weight is on the back leg, only the heel of the opposite foot touches the ground; and when weight is on the forward leg, only the toes of the opposite foot touch the ground. Do not lift the back heel very high, only about one-half inch off the floor.

Ancient Chinese philosophers called the void, which prevailed before the world was created and from which the universe was formed, Wu-Chi or ultimate nothingness. This nothingness was the source of movement and stillness. Yin and Yang and everything in the universe is believed to evolve continually from the unperceivable source. Lao-Tzu called it Tao, the I Ching named it T'ai-Chi and Wang Tsung-Yueh (Ching Dynasty) in his theory of T'ai-Chi Chuan commented:

> *T'ai-Chi is born of Wu-Chi or the ultimate nothingness. It is the origin of dynamic and static states and the mother of Yin and Yang. If they move, they separate. If they remain static, they combine.*

Therefore, the concepts of Wu-Chi and T'ai-Chi describe not only aspects of creation of the universe, but also stages of all relationships between people, between objects and between people and objects.

When something arises from Wu Chi, the state of T'ai-Chi begins. The two aspects then include the voidness of Wu-Chi which is Yin and the something originating from Wu-Chi is Yang. Yin and Yang are complementary opposites which unite to form a whole. However, there is a harmonious relationship between them.

> — From *The Tao of T'ai Chi Chuan, Way to Rejuvenation*[2]

APPENDIX

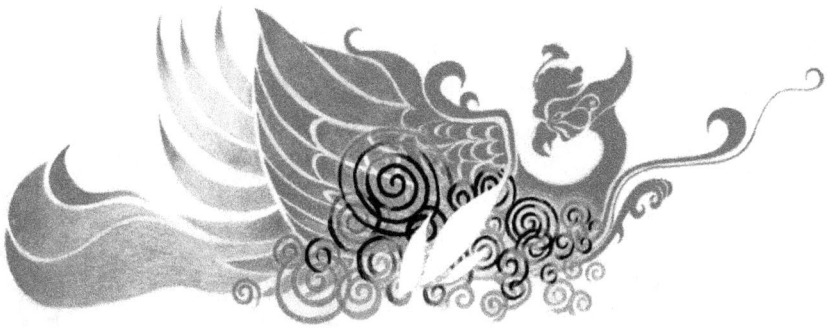

Microcosmic Orbit Meditation[9]
(Often used at end of a *T'ai Chi* session)

太极

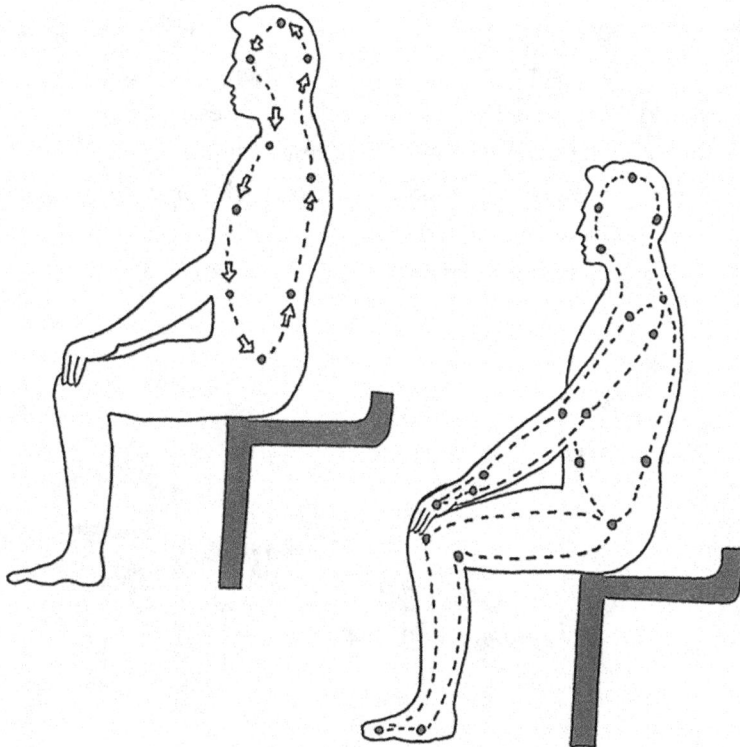

This is a very good meditation for beginning students. Let go of all thoughts and worries. Sit relaxed with spine straight. The Microcosmic Orbit guides the life force so it flows in a loop up the spine and down the front acupuncture channels of the body. Circulating *Chi* in the Microcosmic Orbit assists in counteracting stress.

Sit in a straight chair or cross-legged on the floor. The hands are in front of the lower *tan tien*, the right hand forming a circle with the right thumb and index finger and the thumb of the left hand through this circle. This mudra is called *holding the mind*.

The tongue touches the roof of the palate to complete the circuit of the Governing Channel (back) and the Functional Channel (front). Feel your breath coming in and going out. Start at third eye and inhale down the front and tense the anal muscle, exhale up the back, visualizing the breath going up the spine to the crown. You can see this as a blue mist. When you reach the crown, mentally say the word *hing (hinnnng)*. Pause a few seconds.

Continue inhaling down the front and exhaling up the spine. As you get proficient, you can hold the anal lock for three orbits and then nine orbits. You can practice this for five to ten minutes or longer. When finished, relax with your hands on your legs.

> *T'ai Chi comes from Wu-Chi*
> *And is the mother of yin and yang.*
> *In movement they separate.*
> *In stillness they fuse.*
>
> — Chang San-Feng,
> *T'ai Chi Classics*

History of Microcosmic Orbit

Mantak Chia introduced the "Microcosmic Orbit" to the West in 1983 in *Awaken Healing Energy Through the Tao*. Many believe that before that time much of the Eastern energy practices brought to the West were incomplete because they contained only the ascending *Yang*/masculine channel (which brings the energy up the spine). They did not teach the descending *Yin*/feminine channel of the life-force energy loop. Taoism is one of the oldest spiritual paths to advocate cultivating the feminine to gain balance and wholeness.

Mantak Chia writes, "The Microcosmic Orbit balances and integrates all seven chakras into a single unified chakra ... Rotating *Chi* in the Orbit up the spine and down the front channel regulates the positively and negatively charged points opposite the chakras. I believe these polarities create the minor vortices called chakras, causing them to spin like wheels. By increasing *Chi* flow in the Orbit, the energies flowing through all the chakras are amplified and balanced simultaneously."

Mantak Chia's book, *Healing Light of the Tao—Foundational Practices to Awaken Chi Energy*[10], a sequel, 1993–2008, presents introductory and more advanced methods of *Chi* cultivation with the Microcosmic Orbit, offering a full understanding of Taoist spiritual theory through its comprehensive overview of the complete Taoist body/mind/spirit system. The book also includes more advanced meditation methods for absorbing the higher frequencies of Earth Force, Cosmic Force, and Universal Force (Heavenly *Chi*) into the basic orbit. It establishes a spiritual science that not only emphasizes practical benefits to health, sexual vitality, and emotional balance, but also shows how changes made in the energy body can lead to physical rejuvenation that the Taoists called immortality.

Mantak Chia founded the Universal Healing Tao System in 1979 and is the author of thirty-one books.

Sketches from Lu K'uan Yu's Book,
Taoist Yoga, Alchemy and Immortality[11]

The teachings in this classic text have been preserved for the last 45 centuries instructing readers in the techniques of transforming sexual energy into spiritual consciousness. The author of this classic text in Taoist Yoga is Lu K'uan Yu (Charles Luk). He was born in China in 1898 and devoted himself to presenting many Buddhist texts to preserve Buddhism in the West. These ancient sketches illustrate how far back the teaching of the Microcosmic Orbit goes.

9 THE IMMORTAL BREATHING OR THE SELF-WINDING WHEEL OF THE LAW

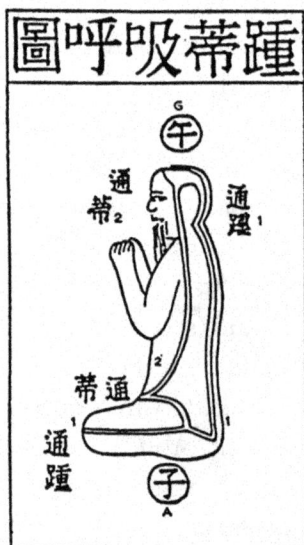

Figure 7 The heel and trunk channels. 1 the heel channel (tung chung) from the heels to the brain. 2 the trunk channel (tung ti) from the lower abdomen to the brain.

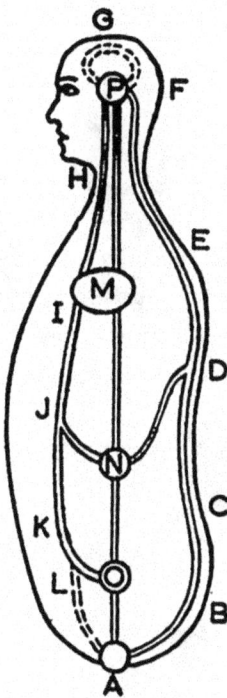

The channel of control (*tu mo*)
A B C D E F:
A (tzu *cardinal point North*—the mortal gate (sheng szu ch'iao)
B (ch'uo) intermediate point
C (yin) intermediate point
D (mao) *cardinal point East*, wood (cleansing)
E (ch'en) intermediate point
F (szu) intermediate point
The channel of function (*jen mo*)
G H I J K L :
G (wu) *cardinal point South*—the brain (ni wan)
H (wei) intermediate point
I (shen) intermediate point
J (yu) *cardinal point West*, metal (purifying)
K (shu) intermediate point
L (hai) intermediate point
The thrusting channel (*ch'ung mo*)
M N O A:
M (li) the heart—house of fire
N (chung t'u) the central earth, the solar plexus (chiang kung)
O (k'an) the lower tan t'ien—house of water
P The centre of the brain(tsu ch'iao)

Figure 8 The channels of control, function and thrusting.

When something arises from Wu-Chi, the state of T'ai-Chi begins. The two aspects then include the voidness of Wu-Chi which is Yin and the something originating from Wu-Chi is Yang. Yin and Yang are complementary opposites which unite to form a whole. However, there is a harmonious relationship between them.

> — Jou, Tsung Hwa., *The Tao of T'ai-Chi Chuan, Way to Rejuvenation*

R.

Cardiovascular System[12]

太極

The deep breathing of *T'ai Chi* regulates the respiratory system, helping to treat respiratory ailments such as asthma, bronchitis and emphysema. The movements stimulate the circulatory, lymphatic and immune systems and the central nervous system.

The cardiovascular system composed of arteries, veins and capillaries circulates the blood, leaving the heart, reaching a body region, distributing nutrients or gases at the capillary level, and then returns it to the heart. The arteries conduct blood away from the heart. The arterial system is a high-pressure system, and the structure of its walls reflects this as they are thicker and more organized than the veins. The smooth muscle layer acts in regulating blood distribution and, in the smaller arteries, may completely resist blood flow into a capillary network.

The veins conduct blood under lower pressure and return it to the heart. They have much less muscle and elastic tissue in their walls and can stretch considerably to become a virtual reservoir of blood in themselves. Valves at certain points in the venous system of the limbs and neck prevent backward flow and resist blood pooling in the lower extremities. The capillaries are simple tubes in which nutrients and gases can diffuse into or from the tissues in response to simple diffusion and osmotic pressure.

The illustration shows only the major arteries. Veins are more numerous than arteries. Usually veins ride with arteries of the same name. The veins receive the tributaries that drain those tissues of deoxygenated blood and the arteries whose branches supply the tissues with oxygenated blood. All blood returns to the right atrium of the heart by way of either the superior or the inferior vena cava except for the coronary and pulmonary blood.

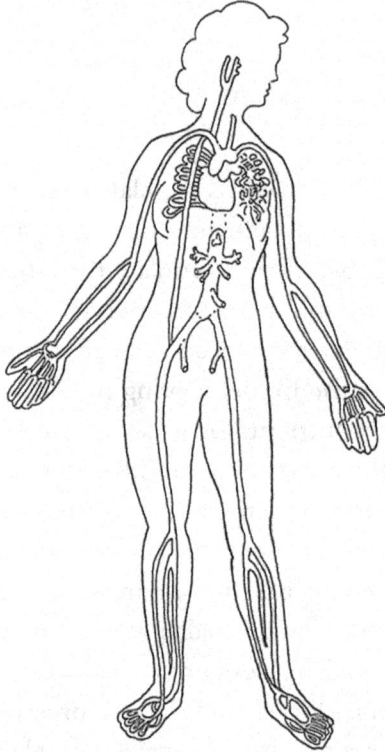

At no point or level of activity in the physical world or in our world of experience are things ever at a standstill. All is action. All is energy. All moves in accord with law. Nothing is changeless. The only thing constant is change, the necessary expression of a creativity which flows from the Mind of the Universe, which is ceaseless in Its action. Power is intrinsically there; we only use and direct It.

— Ernest Holmes, *A New Design for Living*

S.

Lymphatic System[12]

太极

How does *T'ai Chi* exercises benefit immunity and longevity? According to an article by the Cancer Research UK, *T'ai Chi* movements stimulate the lymphatic system and can energize the thymus gland to prevent the creation of T-cells—which prevents cancer from developing. This helps with an aging population as the lymphatic system's immune function deteriorates with age. Doing *T'ai Chi* movements is an excellent way for those who cannot participate in strenuous exercise to keep the lymphatic system healthy.

The body is largely fluid. These fluids require constant circulation, and the pump that maintains this circulation is largely the heart. The heart drives the fluid of the blood's vascular system, and all the other vascular fluids of the body must ultimately return to the vascular system to return to the heart. Veins return blood to the heart, and special fluid "compartments" of the eyes, brain, ears and the lymphatic vessels generally drain into veins.

Arising from veins, the lymphatic vessels are closely associated with veins throughout most parts of the body. They assist veins in their function by drawing from many of the body tissues and increasing the amount of fluid return to the heart.

The lymph vascular network does not form a closed loop system like the blood's vascular system. Lymph vessels begin as tiny, colorless, unconnected capillaries in the connective tissues. These merge to form progressively larger vessels that are interrupted at various sites by small filtering stations called lymph nodes. Looking like small veins, these ducts pour over two quarts of lymph into the brachiocephalic veins every twenty-four hours.

This lymph system has no heart of its own, so lymph flow largely depends upon the kneading action of neighboring skeletal muscles as they alternately contract and relax.

In addition to a network of vessels, the lymphatic system includes a variety of organs. Lymph nodes, along with the spleen, thymus, tonsils, nodules and diffuse lymphatic tissue make up the lymphatic organs. These lymph (filtering) nodes are normally the size of small kidney beans. The cells in the center of the nodes absorb bacteria. These cells strain the lymph. Lymph nodes make up an important part of the body's defense system, and their enlargement may be an indication of an ongoing disease process.

Heaven is enduring. Earth is everlasting. Heaven and earth are infinite in time and space because they do not give birth to themselves. They exist without the consciousness of self. Therefore the sage, the man who flows with Tao, puts his self in the back, and stays in front. By putting his self outside, therefore he exists inside. As in T'ai Chi, the best foot forward really means that we yield back in order to advance. But the sage does not make a conscious effort to put his self last in order to stay in the front. He realizes his self by being selfless.

— Embrace Tiger, Return to Mountain[1]

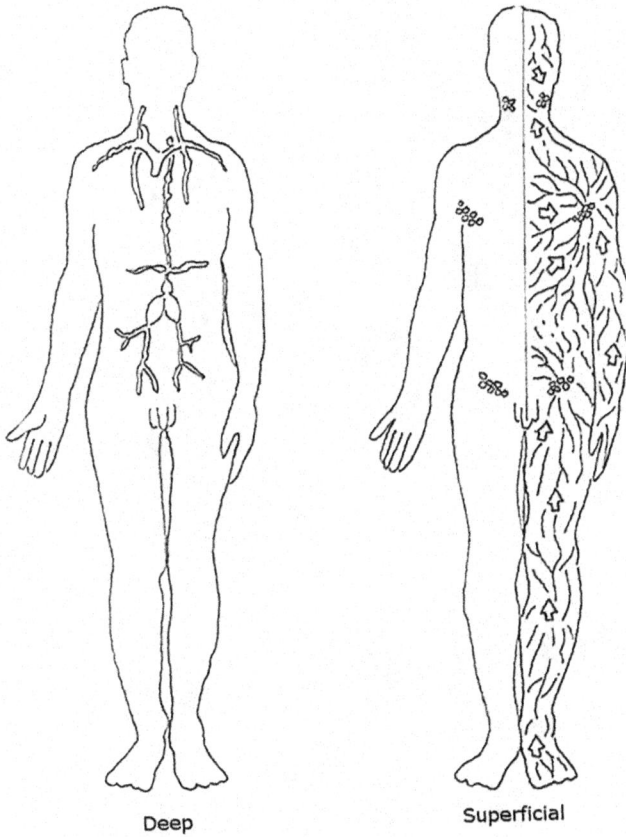

Deep   Superficial

Lymphatic System
Deep and Superficial Channels
of Lymph Drainage

T.

T'ai Chi Books
(only some of many)

太极

Mantak Chia

Awaken Healing Energy Through the Tao: The Taoist Secret of Circulating Internal Power, 1989, originally introducing The Microcosmic Orbit circulating down front and up back.

Taoist Secrets of Love: Cultivating Male Sexual Energy, 1984.

Awaken Healing Energy Through The Tao: The Taoist Secret of Circulating Internal Power, 1983.

Healing Love Through the Tao: Cultivating Female Sexual Energy, 2005.

Healing Light of the Tao, 1993, 2008, Destiny Books.

The Inner Structure of T'ai Chi: Mastering the Classic Form of T'ai Chi Chi Kung, 2005.

Mantak Chia founded the Universal Healing Tao System in 1979 and has been the student of several Taoist masters.

Robert Chuckrow

The T'ai Chi Book: Refining and Enjoying a Lifetime of Practice, 1998. The book introduces beginners to the principles behind *T'ai Chi*. The author introduces complex elements of *T'ai Chi*, how to cultivate and feel *Chi*, how to train mindfulness, and more.

T'ai Chi Walking

T'ai Chi Dynamics

Robert Chuckrow has studied *T'ai Chi, Chi Kung* since 1970 under many masters.

B. K. Frantzis

The Big Book of T'ai Chi: Build Health Fast in Slow Motion, 2003.

Opening the Energy Gates of Your Body: Qigong for Lifelong Health, 1993, 2005. This book has been called a classic that has influenced thousands of Westerners to learn to activate their *Chi* to improve their health, reduce stress and reverse effects of aging.

The Power of Internal Martial Arts and Chi: Combat and Energy Secrets of Ba Gua T'ai Chi and Hsing-I, 1998, 2007. This describes three main internal martial arts—*T'ai Chi, hsing-i* and *ba gua.*

Dragon and Tiger Medical Qigong, Volume 1: Develop Health and Energy in 7 Simple Movements, 2010. This *qigong* has been practiced in China to release stress and maintain robust health and has also been used to prevent and heal cancer.

The CHI Revolution: Harnessing the Healing Power of Your Life Force, 2008. Frantzis challenges readers to embark on an inner revolution to reclaim joy and happiness in life, reverse the effects of aging and release their stress and negative emotions.

Frantzis has forty years of training in ancient Chinese practices.

Roger Jahnke

The Healing Promise of Qi: Creating Extraordinary Wellness Through Qigong and T'ai Chi, 2002. The author is an internationally respected doctor of Chinese medicine and author of the bestselling *The Healer Within*. He explains the concepts of *Qi Gong* in practical terms. The book has 125 illustrations and describes many simple *Qi Gong* tools, practices, and techniques for utilizing the incredible power of *qi*.

Dr. Paul Lam

T'ai Chi for Beginners and the 24 Forms, 2006. It provides an easy step-by-step guide to an enjoyable form of exercise that will improve your general well-being.

T'ai Chi for Arthritis

T'ai Chi Music

Dr. Lam is a *T'ai Chi* Master and Family Physician in Australia and teaches *T'ai Chi* for health, wellness and longevity.

Waysun Liao

T'ai Chi Classics, 1977, 1990, Shambhala

Restoring Your Life Energy, 2012, Shambhala

Chi—Discovering Your Life Energy, 2009, Shambhala.

The Essence of T'ai Chi, 2007, Shambhala.

T'ai Chi Classics, 2000.

Master Waysun Liao studied *T'ai Chi* in central Taiwan before coming to the United States, where he has taught *T'ai Chi* for thirty years. He also practices herbal medicine, acupuncture and feng-shui. According to Master Liao, the great power of *T'ai Chi* cannot be realized without knowing its inner meaning. *T'ai Chi Classics* presents the inner meaning and techniques of the movements through translations of three core classics, often considered the *"T'ai Chi* Bible."* He is the founder of one of the oldest *T'ai Chi* centers in

North America, in Oak Park, Illinois. The texts are introduced by three chapters explaining how to incrase inner energy (*Ch'i*), transform it into inner power (*jing*), and project this inner power outward to repel an opponent without physical contact. He has taught in the United States for over thirty years.

Benjamin P. Lo, Editor

The Essence of T'ai Chi Ch'uan: The Literary Tradition, 1993, North Atlantic Books, "A handbook of the classical Chinese literature on which the art of *T'ai Chi* is based. First English translation of the classic texts of *T'ai Chi Ch'uan*. This is required reading for practitioners of every style."

Justin Stone

T'ai Chi Chih! Joy Thru Movement, 2009. This photo-text has complete instruction for the simple twenty meditative movements. The movements affect the inner organs as well as the muscular structure. Also included are essays on the background and philosophy of the *T'ai Chih Chih* movements. This discipline circulates and balances our internal energy (*Chi*) helping alleviate stress, improving relaxation, health and creativity. Justin has a CD, *T'ai Chi Chih! Joy Thru Movement*, where he discusses its origins and philosophy, what you can experience with regular practice. A DVD by the same name is also available.

Peter M. Wayne, Ph.D., with Mark L. Fuerst

The Harvard Medical School Guide to T'ai Chi—12 Weeks to a Healthy Body, Strong Heart & Sharp Mind, 2013, Shambhala. The author is a *T'ai Chi* teacher and a researcher at Harvard Medical School where he has designed programs for people of all ages. The research highlights fascinating insight into underlying physiological mechanisms that explain how *T'ai Chi* works.

The Harvard Medical School Guide to T'ai Chi is a significant milestone in the integration of Eastern and Western medicine. It deftly summarizes the scientific evidence for the healing potential of this traditional Chinese system of body movement and gives readers practical advice for using it in everyday life. I recommend it highly.
> — Andrew Weil, MD, author of *8 Weeks to Optimum Health*, Professor of Medicine, University of Arizona

Evidence has shown that unhealthy lifestyle is the cause of most if not all chronic conditions such as diabetes, arthritis, and heart disease. Dr. Wayne's book, with his expertise in medical research and T'ai Chi, is a significant step towards modernizing T'ai Chi—essential to making T'ai Chi a central part of practical and effective solutions to the epidemic of chronic disease.
> — Dr. Paul Lam, Director of The *T'ai Chi* for Health Institute and author of *Teaching T'ai Chi Effectively* and *T'ai Chi for Beginners*

U.

T'ai Chi and *Gigong*
Websites

太极

In a Google search when you enter "Health benefits of Tai Chi" almost 500 websites will come up. A sampling follows:

Mayo Clinic:

www.mayoclinic.com

An article titled "Tai Chi: A gentle way to fight stress—Tai Chi helps reduce stress and anxiety. And it also helps increase flexibility and balance" (www.mayoclinic.com/health/tai-chi/SA00087) explores: What is t'ai chi? Who can do t'ai chi, Why try t'ai chi? How to get started with t'ai chi and maintaining the benefits of t'ai chi.

> "If you're looking for a way to reduce stress, consider t'ai chi (TIE-CHEE). Originally developed for self-defense, t'ai chi has evolved into a graceful form of exercise that's now used for stress reduction and a variety of other health conditions. Often described as meditation in motion, t'ai chi promotes serenity through gentle, flowing movements."

SFQ—Spring Forest Qigong:
www.springforestqigong.com

This website has a wealth of information.

"Spring Forest Qigong (pronounced 'chee gong') is a simple, efficient, and effective method for helping you experience your optimal health, wellness, and happiness; helping you heal physical and emotional pain; and enhancing the quality of your life and the lives of others.

SFQ is comprised of four parts that all work together:
- Breathing
- Gentle movements (active exercises)
- Mental focus
- Sound

Helpful Tips:
- Breathe slowly, gently, deeply
- Let your body relax
- Focus on feeling the energy
- Do these movements standing, sitting or lying down …

Master Chunyi Lin designed all Spring Forest *Qigong* active exercises to enhance the flow of your energy, open any energy blockages you may have, and bring your energy back into balance.

Having balanced, smoothly-flowing energy is the key to experiencing and maintaining your optimal health and wellness."

T'ai Chi for Beginners, 8 Lessons with Dr. Paul Lam—free first lesson:
www.youtube.com/watch?v=hIOHGrYCEJ4

Dr. Lam explains about *T'ai Chi*, its benefits and some general instructions. In this 44-minute video, he explains it is better to learn a few movements and do them well.

service@taichiproductions.com

World T'ai Chi & Qigong (Chi Kung) Day:
www.worldtaichiday.org/Weblinks.html

Listed are hundred of links to *T'ai Chi* and *Qigong* websites, organized by local or general information. You can search in the United States by your state or city to find contact information for schools or teachers.

Some of the topics covered: Curious About *T'ai Chi* and *Qigong?* Beginner-Enthusiast Resources, Teacher-School Resources and Tools, Be a Part of a Global Health & Healing Event, TCM, Acupuncture, Medical Research, DVDs, Books, *Qigong* Machines, Chinese Herbs, etc.

World *T'ai Chi* and *Qigong* Day takes place the last Saturday of April each year. The United Nations Recognizes World *T'ai Chi* and *Qigong* Day.

WholeHealthMD.com
www.wholehealthmd.com

Physician-directed health information combining conventional medicine and alternative therapies to improve health. Health Benefits: Arthritis, Balance, Circulation problems, High blood pressure, Multiple Sclerosis, Stress.

T'ai Chi Chih Community:
www.tcccommunity.net and www.taichichih.org

The TCC community of teachers is led by Sr. Antonia Cooper, current guide.

> "T'ai Chi Chih® (TCC) was originated in 1974 by
> American T'ai Chi Master, Justin Stone, in
> Albuquerque, New Mexico. Motivated by his work in
> teaching T'ai Chi Chuan and other disciplines, over a
> period of several years, Justin Stone refined the
> movements we use today in T'ai Chi Chih® and
> introduced them to students in the Albuquerque,
> New Mexico area."

Harvard Health Publications—Harvard Medical School:
www.health.harvard.edu

Enter *Tai Chi* in the Advanced Search and you can bring up many articles on the benefits of *Tai Chi*:

> "The health benefits of tai chi"
> "Try tai chi to improve balance, avoid falls"
> "Tai chi improves balance and motor control in
> Parkingson's disease"
> "Tai chi eases several medical conditions"
> "Best exercise for balance"
> "Mindfulness meditation improves connections in
> the brain"

Publications:

T'ai Chi & Alternative Health Magazine, United Kingdom:
www.taichiwl.demon.co.uk/tcah.html

Qigong Institute Newsletter:
www.qigonginstitute.org/main_page/main_page.php

Taijiquan Journal:
www.taijiquanjournal.com

T'ai Chi Magazine:
www.tai-chi.com

The International Magazine of T'ai Chi Chuan has been serving the *T'ai Chi* community since 1977. It covers *T'ai Chi Chuan*, *qigong*, and other internal martial arts and similar Chinese disciplines which contribute to fitness, health and well-being. The articles also have interviews with experts about the philosophy behind internal martial arts.

WorldTaiChiDay.org—The Official Online World T'ai Chi & Qigong Day News Magazine:
www.worldtaichiday.org/Associations.html

You are able to stay up-to-date with all things *T'ai Chi* and *Qigong* with the *T'ai Chi and Qigong Day Ezine Magazine* and it is free. Check out the history, philosophy, modern science research, Tips on Teaching or Learning *T'ai Chi & Qigong*, Healthy Recipes and more. This ezine can be translated into 39 languages.

National and International *T'ai Chi* or *Qigong* Associations:

American Qigong Association:
www.eastwestqi.com/aqa—Promote *Qigong*, bringing it into the mainstream as a health practice.

Canadian Taijiquan Federation:
www.canadiantaijiquanfederation.ca

Healing Tao USA (and Healing Tao University):
www.HealingTaoUSA.com—Medical and Spiritual Qigong: Healthy Exercise DVDs, Primordial *T'ai Chi*: Open a Loving Heart, Tao Sexual Inner Alchemy: Feel Your Bliss.

Institute of Integral *Qigong* and *T'ai Chi*:
www.HealerWithin.com—Healer Within Community.

National Qigong Association:
www.nqa.org

Northwest T'ai Chi Chuan Association:
www.dotaichi.com—Tchoung Ta-Tchen's Dual Style *T'ai Chi*.

Practice for Health and Vitality:
www.FeeltheQi.com—Mind-Body-Spirit Transformation with *T'ai Chi* and *Qigong*—Dr. Roger Jahnke.

The Qigong Institute:
www.qigonginstitute.org—Promoting *Qigong* and Energy Medicine through Research and Education

T'ai Chi Chih Association:

www.taichichihassociation.org

Included are TCC Events, free guided TCC Practice and Video clips of Justin Stone demonstrating: Pulling Taffy and Variations, Six Healing Sounds, Joyous Breath, Light at the Top of the Head/Light at the Temple, Passing Clouds, Working the Pulley. Also listed are four articles on the Benefits from Practicing *T'ai Chi Chih*.

T'ai Chi Healthways:

www.taichihealthways.com—Authoritative *T'ai Chi* and *Qigong* in San Diego.

Unique Healing Solutions:

www.uniquehealingsolutions.com—Provides videos, workshops and natural healing products, *Qigong*, to promote holistic health, prevention and anti-aging.

Wu (Hao) Taijiquan Association USA:

www.wuhaotaichi.com—Traditional *T'ai Chi*—Lifetime Health and Fitness.

V.

Research Articles on the Benefits of Doing *T'ai Chi*

太极

What is this phenomenon the past few years mentioned in many of the articles on the benefits of doing *T'ai Chi*? For thousands of years, it was a sacred practice known only to a few. Then it was introduced into the west.

Historically, it is a wonderful discipline for your health and sense of well-being. It is a spiritual discipline as well. Science and the medical profession now have researched many of the benefits derived from doing the movements. And people find them fun to do. Actually, the more you do the lovely dance-like movements, you discover the health benefits are cumulative.

The practice has been looked upon by some spas and health clubs as a means to make money. Unfortunately, in some cases, the practice has been marginalized, teaching *T'ai Chi* or *Qigong* has become an industry and this has bothered some purists. Chinese masters are probably rolling over in their graves. It used to be a deep experience for the lucky few who practiced it. Mastering some of the 70,000 or more different forms of *Qigong* can take decades.

1. "The Healing Power of Tai Chi Chuan—Ancient Art Can Cure Many Maladies," by Frank Petrillo Jr., *Black Belt Magazine*, November, 1992, pp. 54-7.

2. In July 31, 2002, an article in *Time Magazine* is titled "Why T'ai Chi is the Perfect Exercise." The author, Christine Gorman, writes that *T'ai Chi* combines intense mental focus with deliberate, graceful movements that improve strength, agility and balance. She sites that scientists at the Oregon Research Institute in Eugene reported that *T'ai Chi* offers the greatest benefit to older men and women who are healthy but inactive. The regular practice helps reduce falls and the goal is to go at your own pace and that "pain is no gain."

T'ai Chi plus walking is a good combination for well-being. Younger people need aerobic activity in addition but can benefit from *T'ai Chi's* capacity to reduce stress. A big plus is that people enjoy doing *T'ai Chi.*

3. In May 13, 2003 an article in *The Wall Street Journal* by Jane Spencer is titled "The Next Yoga: A Sweat-Free Workout, Giving Up on Perfect Pecs, Boomers Embrace Qigong; Tiger Woods's Secret Weapon?" The ancient practice of Qigong is showing up alongside yoga and aqua aerobics as the hottest trend in stress relief at American spas and health clubs for housewives, models and stockbrokers.

The practice has been done in China and Tibet for over four thousand years. The Chinese peasants used qigong to manage daily stresses of invading barbarians. Now posh gyms like the Sports Club/LA have classes such as "SynerChi Sculpt" which combines qigong, yoga and weightlifting. The Spa at Turnberry Isle in Aventura, Florida has added *qigong* to its activity schedule. Employees at companies like Prudential Financial and Mattel have taken *gigong* workshops and golf pros are rushing to take private lessons after hearing rumors that Tiger Woods is practicing it.

One of the fitness gurus says that they are bringing these beautiful movements to the mainstream. The baby boomers are realizing they don't need to bounce around as much to achieve fitness. They want a more holistic approach. Baby boomers are the fastest growing segment of gym members and ten percent of all Americans over the age of 55 that belong to a health club.

4. **T'ai Chi Benefits Chronic Conditions:** United States and Canadian scientists have reviewed four dozen studies in North America, Australia and Asia. They have reached interesting conclusions regarding the ancient art of *T'ai Chi*. Their analysis was published in *Archives of Internal Medicine* and reported in *Acupuncture Today*, July 2004. The article was titled "T'ai Chi: Good for the Mind, Good for the Body." They researched English and Chinese language articles regarding the practice of *T'ai Chi* published between 1963 and April 2002.

The scientists reported that for elderly people with chronic diseases, practicing *T'ai Chi* offers many physical and mental benefits. The majority of the studies found a wide range of positive benefits on overall health and well-being, from increased muscle strength and flexibility, to lowered blood pressure, to enhanced immune function.

Balance control and falls: Eleven studies measured postural stability, strength, flexibility and other aspects of a person's ability to maintain balance. Long-term practitioners had greater flexibility in the lower extremities and *T'ai Chi* improved one's gait.

Cardiovascular and respiratory systems: A dozen studies with patients of various ages and doing several styles of *T'ai Chi* found that elderly patients who practiced four times a week for one year had improved cardio-respiratory function, strength and flexibility.

Endocrine and immune systems: Practicing *T'ai Chi* improved endocrine function in one study of 98 elderly men. Another study found that regularly practicing for four years, resulted in a larger number of a class of immune cells called T-cells in the blood.

Hypertension: Four studies of more than 400 patients practicing *T'ai Chi* from 8 weeks to 3 years found reductions in systolic blood pressure.

Musculoskeletal conditions: Of four studies, one group of patients practiced *T'ai Chi* for 12 weeks had improved arthritic symptoms, decreased tension and greater satisfaction with general health. One study suggested that *T'ai Chi* could improve muscle strength and endurance in the knees of elderly people and a fourth study with patients with multiple sclerosis reported patients practicing *T'ai Chi* had improvements in vitality, social functioning, and mental health.

Psychological responses: Of six studies, two demonstrated that older participants participating in a *T'ai Chi* program showed better scores that measured depression, psychological distress and positive well-being. Another study showed participants with Alzheimer's disease who practiced *T'ai Chi* twice a week for seven weeks demonstrated "thinking that was focused and insightful, beyond the level normally manifested for this group of participants."

"All the indications from this review show *T'ai Chi* is beneficial. But we cannot yet draw scientific conclusions," Wang added that she and her colleagues would soon embark on a new study to determine why *T'ai Chi* works, and which patients can get the most benefits from it.

References:
Wang C, Collet JP, Lau J. "The effect of T'ai Chi on health outcomes in patients with chronic conditions. A systematic review." *Archives of Internal Medicine*, March 8, 2004.

5. An article titled "The Health Benefits of Tai Chi," Harvard Medical School, dated May 1, 2009, lists benefits in muscle strength, flexibiliity, balance, and aerobic conditioning.

Muscle strength. A study published in 2006 in *Alternative Therapies in Health and Medicine* by Stanford University reported benefits after 36 classes in 12 weeks. The group of men and women showed improvement in both lower body and upper body strength. The participants also boosted upper and lower body *flexibility.*

Arthritis. In October 2008, Tufts University did a 40-person study of an hour of *T'ai Chi* twice a week for 12 weeks. It resulted in reduced pain and improved mood and physical functioning in comparison to standard stretching exercises.

Low bone density. Six controlled studies by Harvard researchers showed that T'ai Chi may be a safe and effective way to maintain bone density in postmenopausal women.

Breast cancer. A 2008 study at the University of Rochester (published in *Medicine and Sport Science*) found that that the quality of life improved in women with breast cancer after a 12-week program of *T'ai Chi.* This included aerobic capacity, muscular strength and flexibility.

Heart disease. In September 2008, the *Journal of Alternative and Complementary Medicine* reported a 53-person study at the National Taiwan University. It stated that after a year of *T'ai Chi*, it boosted exercise capacity, lowered blood pressure, improved levels of cholesterol, triglycerides, insulin and C-reactive protein in people at higher risk for heart disease.

Heart failure. At Harvard Medical School, in a 30-person pilot study, 12 weeks of *T'ai Chi* improved the participants' ability to walk and quality of life and also reducing blood levels of B-type natriuretic protein.

Hypertension. In *Preventive Cardiology*, Spring 2008, Dr. Yeh reports on a review of 26 studies in English or Chinese. In 85% of trials, *T'ai Chi* lowered blood pressure.

Parkinson's disease. In October 2008, the Washington University School of Medicine in St. Louis, published in *Gait and Posture* a 33-person pilot study. It found that people with mild to moderately severe Parkinson's disease showed improved balance, walking ability, and overall well-being after 20 *T'ai Chi* sessions.

Sleep problems. In the July 2008 issue of the journal Sleep, at University of California, Los Angeles had a study of 112 healthy older adults with moderate sleep complaints. After 16 weeks of *T'ai Chi*, the quality and duration of sleep improved.

Stroke. In the January 2009 issue of Neurorehabilitation and Neural Repair, a study was published of 136 patients who had a stroke at least six months earlier. After 12 weeks of *T'ai Chi*, there was improved standing balance.

Harvard Medical School concludes:

> "This gentle form of exercise can prevent or ease
> many ills of aging and could be the perfect activity
> for the rest of your life. T'ai Chi is often described
> as 'meditation in motion,' but it might be called
> 'medication in motion.' It originated in China as a
> martial art, and there is growing evidence that this
> mind-body practice has value in treating or
> preventing many health problems. The movements
> are usually circular and never forced; the muscles are
> relaxed and the joints are not fully extended or bent
> and connective tissues are not stretched. T'ai Chi can

be adapted for anyone from the most fit to people confined to wheelchairs."

An assistant professor of medicine at Harvard Medical School, Peter M. Wayne, has stated that there is a growing body of carefully conducted research in building a case for using *T'ai Chi* along with standard medical treatment for the prevention and rehabilitation of many conditions associated with age.

Many of the forms have names in honor of the people who devised the sets of movements which are called forms, i.e. *Yang*, *Wu*, and *Cheng*. The different movements often have names of animals. *T'ai Chi* is slow and gentle and doesn't leave you breathless. It does address the key components of fitness, i.e., muscle strength, flexibility, balance, and to a lesser degree aerobic condition.

www.health.harvard.edu/staying-healthy/the-health-benefits-of-tai-chi

6. On July 1, 2010, the National Center for Complementary and Alternative Medicine published an article, "T'ai Chi and Qi Gong Show Some Beneficial Health Effects" referred to the researchers from the Institute of Integral Qigong and T'ai Chi. They concluded that evidence is sufficient to suggest that *T'ai Chi* and *Qigong* are a viable alternative to conventional forms of exercise.

7. In August 31, 2010, one of the most extensive reviews of the research literature on the health benefits of *T'ai Chi* and *Qigong* was published. This review presents the entire *Qigong* and *T'ai Chi* "evidence base" in one comprehensive presentation. It was conducted by The Institute of Integral *Qigong* and *T'ai Chi* (a training division of Health Action, Inc., in Santa Barbara, California) in collaboration with Arizona State University and the

University of Arizona. This review was published in the *American Journal of Health Promotion (AJHP)*.

The Chinese have been doing these practices for thousands of years. Now, there is an "evidence base" for *Qigong* and *T'ai Chi* emerging from within the Western world's scientific framework.

This recent collaboration to review the *Qigong* and *T'ai Chi* literature has resulted in the most comprehensive review of the research literature on *Qigong* and *T'ai Chi* that has ever been produced. Dr. Roger Jahnke, OMD and his colleague, Dr. Linda Larkey, applied a rigorous criterion wherein only the best randomized controlled trials were considered in the review. The total of such research between 1993 and the end of 2007 was an impressive 77 trials.

The total number of study participants was 6,410 with the highest number of studies of 27 addressing psychological issues. Cardiac studies numbered 23 and falls prevention trials numbered 19. Other areas of positive influence included bone density, immune capacity, quality of life and physical function.

Drs. Jahke and Larkey concluded that, "with the mounting evidence for health benefits and the current progress in research methodology, it is likely that T'ai Chi and Qigong will play a strong role in the emerging integrative medicine system as well as in prevention based interventions in the evolving health care delivery system." The importance of the article was so significant that it was reviewed on ABC News. Dr. Timithy Jones on a short video: "Eastern Exercises Stand the Test of Time."

Dr. Roger Jahke, from the Institute of Integral Qigong and T'ai Chi, concludes that cultivating the *Qi* through Integral *Qigong* and *T'ai Chi* triggers numerous health benefits:

1. *Qigong* and *T'ai Chi* initiate the "relaxation response," which is fostered when the mind is freed from its many distractions. This decreases the sympathetic function of the autonomic nervous

system, which in turn reduces heart rate and blood pressure, dilates the blood capillaries, and optimizes the delivery of oxygen and nutrition to the tissues.

2. *Qigong* and *T'ai Chi* alter the neurochemistry profile toward accelerated inner healing function.

3. *Qigong* and *T'ai Chi* enhance the efficiency of the immune system through increased rate and flow of the lymphatic fluid and activation of immune cells.

4. *Qigong* and *T'ai Chi* increases the efficiency of cell metabolism and tissue regeneration through increased circulation of oxygen and nutrient rich blood to the brain, organs and tissues.

5. *Qigong* and *T'ai Chi* coordinate and balance right/left brain hemisphere dominance promoting deeper sleep, reduced anxiety and mental clarity.

6. *Qigong* and *T'ai Chi* induce alpha and, in some cases, theta brain waves which reduce heart rate and blood pressure, facilitating relaxation, and mental focus; this optimizes the body's self-regulative mechanisms by decreasing the activity of the sympathetic nervous system.

7. *Qigong* and *T'ai Chi* moderate the function of the hypothalamus, pituitary, and pineal glands, as well as the cerebrospinal fluid system of the brain and spinal cord, which manages pain and mood as well as optimizing immune function.

To request a copy of the entire article, "Health Benefits of *T'ai Chi* and *Qigong*," email Dr. Roger Jahnke at info@iiqtc.org.

Titles by Dr. Roger Jahnke:

The Healing Promise of Qi: Creating Extraordinary Wellness Through Qigong and T'ai Chi (Book)

Qigong-Chi Kung: Awakening and Mastering the Medicine Within You (DVD)

Essentials of Qigong: The Ancient Chinese Way to Better Health (DVD)

(See article No. 23—March 2015)

"When people learn about the Healer Within themselves and then take action to care for their own physical, mental, emotional and spiritual health, they are transformed."

— from *The Healer Within* by Dr. Roger Jahnke

8. *U.S. News and World Report*: "For Health Benefits, Try T'ai Chi," by Courtney Rubin, November 26, 2010—"Relief for Fibromyalgia Pain: a Dose of T'ai Chi."

"**Flexibility and strength.** T'ai Chi is credited with so many pluses, physiological and psychological, that Chenchen Wang, an associate professor of medicine at Tufts University, set out earlier this year to analyze 40 studies on it in English and Chinese journals. Wang found that T'ai Chi did indeed promote balance, flexibility, cardiovascular fitness, and strength. In a study comparing it with brisk walking and resistance training, a T'ai Chi group improved more than 30 percent in lower-body strength and 25 percent in arm strength, nearly as much as a weight-training group and more than the walkers. 'Benefit was also found for pain, stress, and anxiety in healthy subjects,' adds Wang, who was influenced by her mother, a Chinese doctor, to study an integration of complementary and alternative medicine with Western medicine."

9. "A Top Ten List of T'ai Chi and Qigong in 2010," Dec. 29, 2010, by Violet Li, *T'ai Chi Examiner.*

Violet Li is an award winning journalist, a 12th generation Chen Style *T'ai Chi* Inheritor, certified *Taiji Taichi*) instructor. She has studied *Taiji, Qigong (Chi Gong)*, and heart fitness with many grandmasters and experts. She has taught *Taichi* and *Chi Gong*. Her passion for *T'ai Chi, Qigong* and fitness motivates her to write articles on the related events. Violet writes locally for the St. Louis *T'ai Chi Examiner.* Please contact her at violet.li@tadi.com

T'ai Chi/Qigong Examiner has been propelled from a local St. Louis (MO) site and spun off to a national site. Additionally, both St. Louis *T'ai Chi/Qigong* site and the National *T'ai Chi/Qigong* site have been fed to other sites. Furthermore, the National *T'ai Chi/Qigong* site has been featured in the national category and three of its articles were on the "front page" of the National Examiner site.

The World Congress on *Qigong* and the Traditional Chinese Medicine (TCM), founded by Dr. Effie Chow, aligned its annual convention date with the *World T'ai Chi & Qigong* Day (WTCQD) this year to jointly celebrate the *T'ai Chi* and *Qigong* world-wide with greater momentum (read Twelfth World Congress on *Qigong* & TCM).

The Center of *Taiji* and *Qigong* was featured in International Exercise Therapy Symposium in October. The International Exercise Therapy Symposium was held in conjunction with the annual Mayo Clinic-Karolinska Institute Conference and the Frontiers of Medicine Program, jointly sponsored by the Mayo Clinic, the Karolinska Institute of Sweden, and the University of Minnesota. This signified that *T'ai Chi/Qigong* is now widely viewed as an important therapy. International Exercise Therapy Symposium will feature Center for *Taiji* & *Qigong* for more information.

A first short movie about *T'ai Chi* (*Final Weapon*) in English, starring Master Ren Guangyi, premiered and awarded at the

International Film Festival in Pasadena, California on July 24, 2010 and continues to get rave reviews in other film festivals. This movie was written and directed by Stephan Berwick, a Western pioneer of Chinese martial arts, actor in the Hong Kong action film of the 1980s, and senior *T'ai Chi* instructor/writer. The significance of this movie is to restore the honor and integrity of the ancient old Chinese martial art of *T'ai Chi*. It also got a rave review at the Coney Island Film Festival.

A first English novel based on *T'ai Chi* and *Qigong* theory is: *2012: The Awakening* by Bill Douglas was published in August. Based on facts, this novel illuminates why it is important to bring the *Yin* energy to the world. Bill also highlights the benefits of practicing *T'ai Chi* and *Qigong* with an engrossing plot. This inspirational thriller has been getting wide-spread attention from the media and spiritual community.

Perhaps the most important event of 2010 was the publication of the English version of Chinese Medical *Qigong* in early Spring. Tianjun Liu, OMD of Beijing University of Chinese Medicine was the Editor in Chief. Dr. Kevin Chen of University of Maryland School of Medicine was Associate Editor in Chief and in charge of the massive translation effort of this textbook. *Qigong Study in Chinese Medicine* is the only official textbook of medical *Chi Gong* in China. It is a collaborative effort of more than thirty faculty members of a dozen top-ranked colleges and universities of the Traditional Chinese Medicine (TCM). The translation effort took four years to complete with 23 outstanding scientists in the Board from China and abroad. The content is rich and extensive. It is a monumental accomplishment to promoting understanding and study of *Qigong* and Traditional Chinese Medicine in the western world.

10. From an article titled "Tai Chi for falls prevention," Feb. 21, 2011, at NHS Networks:

> "The latest research has shown that fear of falling increases the risk of falling. It is also a classic phobic responce so how can tai chi & Chi-kung help?
>
> The answer is in three areas:
> Proprioception – body's ability to sense movement within joints and joint position
> Kinaesthetic awareness - Understanding and sensing where your body is in an open space
> Mindfulness – paying attention to the here and now; feeding into the above two mentioned areas
>
> Fears occur because of future pacing of thoughts (like little in-head movies) that make worst case scenarios seems really real rather than just possible. Mindfulness prevents future pacing because it is only based in the now. Even CBT (cognitive behavioural therapy) has taken this on as a therapeutic tool.
>
> The wonder of tai chi is it has all three of these areas by design, and not as additions, therefore they are a natural process to follow."

www.networks.nhs.uk/nhs-networks/tai-chi-chi-kung-for-rehabilitation/tai-chi-for-falls-prevention

11. In November 3, 2011, an article published in *Prevention Magazine* by Marianne McGinnis, "T'ai Chi: The No-Sweat Way to Boost Immunity."

> "To keep sick days at bay, trade your vitamin C in for a dose of T'ai Chi. It's cheaper, more effective (reving

up your body's disease-fighting defenses by as much as 47%), and even triples the protection you get from a flu shot. The secret to T'ai Chi's elixir-like quality, scientists suspect, lies in its slow movements and controlled breathing. T'ai Chi then marshals the power of both to fight germs. It also zaps stress and helps you to sleep better—both key to a healthy immune system."

www.prevention.com/fitness/fitness-tips/boost-your-immune-system-naturally-tai-chi#ixzz2GORkRGlD

12. In a November 24, 2011 article in Health Day, "T'ai Chi May Provide Arthritis Relief." After two months of practicing *T'ai Chi*, stiffness, fatigue, balance and well-being were improved. The study's lead author, Leigh F. Callahan, an associate professor of medicine at the University of North Carolina at Chapel Hill School of Medicine said, "It reduced pain, stiffness and fatigue, and improved their balance ... Patients also reported gaining a better sense of physical stability. They were able to extend their reach while maintaining their balance, an important feat for people with arthritis ... T'ai Chi has become a lot more mainstream."

The article stated that "T'ai Chi is a form of mind-body exercise, originating as a martial art in China. It utilizes slow gentle movements along with deep breathing and relaxation to build strength and flexibility."

In the study of 247 people, all female and white, which were diagnosed with various types of arthritis, attended one-hour classes, twice a week for two months. The participants were from twenty locations in New Jersey and North Carolina. They said they felt mildly to moderately better and had an improved sense of well-being, and slept better. There was evidence that doing the *T'ai Chi* reduced symptoms of knee arthritis, but not rheumatoid arthritis.

Dr. Callahan, "T'ai Chi appears to provide both physical and mental benefits. The whole program is designed to help people be relaxed and think about their breathing and think about their movements. Everything is slow, deliberate and purposeful."

13."T'ai Chi Improves Symptoms of Parkinson's Disease," CBS News, February 9, 2012, *T'ai Chi*, a type of exercise that guides the body through gentle, flowing poses, may help some of the worst physical problems of Parkinson's disease, a new study shows.

Summary of article:
T'ai Chi Comes Out Tops

For the study, doctors assigned 195 people with mild-to-moderate Parkinson's disease to one of three groups: The first took *T'ai Chi* classes, the second exercised with weights, and the third was assigned to a program of seated stretching. All the groups met for 60-minute sessions twice each week. After six months, people who had been taking *T'ai Chi* were able to lean farther forward or backward without stumbling or falling compared to those who had been doing resistance training or stretching. They were also better able to smoothly direct their movements. And they were able to take longer strides than people in the other two groups. Like resistance training, *T'ai Chi* helped people walk more swiftly, get up from a chair more quickly, and increased leg strength.

14. "T'ai Chi and Postural Stability in Patients with Parkinson's Disease," *The New England Journal of Medicine*, February 9, 2012. Background: Patients with Parkinson's disease have substantially impaired balance, leading to diminished functional ability and an

increased risk of falling. Although exercise is routinely encouraged by health care providers, few programs have been proven effective.

Their conclusions are: "Tai chi training appears to reduce balance impairments in patients with mild-to-moderate Parkinson's disease, with additional benefits of improved functional capacity and reduced falls."

15. "T'ai Chi: A gentle way to fight stress," September 28, 2012, by Mayo Clinic Staff.

> "If you're looking for a way to reduce stress, consider T'ai Chi (TIE-CHEE). Originally developed for self-defense, T'ai Chi has evolved into a graceful form of exercise that's now used for stress reduction and a variety of other health conditions. Often described as meditation in motion, T'ai Chi promotes serenity through gentle, flowing movements."

The Mayo Clinic staff reported that doing a series of *T'ai Chi* movements is a gentle way to fight stress. They report that *T'ai Chi* promotes serenity through the gentle, flowing movements and that it can be a positive part of an overall approach to improving your health. Benefits they list are decreased stress and anxiety, increased aerobic capacity, increased energy and stamina, increased flexibility, balance and agility; and increased muscle strength and definition. Mayo Clinic recommends continuing *T'ai Chi* after a 12-week *T'ai Chi* class in order to obtain greater benefits.

(See article No. 19—May 18, 2013)

16. A news story, "Tai chi and heart health in older people," in the *Daily Mail* on April 5, 2012 reports that *doing T'ai Chi can boost elderly people's hearts*. People who practiced regularly had more elasticity in their arteries and greater muscle strength in their knees. They state that there is much research demonstrating heart and health benefits of *T'ai Chi* for people with arthritis or those at risk of falling.

The study was done by researchers from The Hong Kong Polytechnic University and the University of Illinois, USA.

17. In June 19, 2012, an article published in the *Journal of Alzheimer's Disease* reported that *T'ai Chi increases brain size* from a trial of Chinese elderly. Scientists were from the University of South Florida and Fudan University in Shanghai. Findings were based on an 8-month controlled trial. An overview article titled "Tai Chi increases brain size and benefits cognition in randomized controlled trial of Chinese elderly" can be found at the University of South Florida Health News website.

18. In June 17, 2013, Reuters (U.S Edition), had an article, "T'ai Chi: getting there more slowly, but gracefully and intact." T'ai Chi as become a staple in senior citizen centers and in dawn sightings in public parks. The article states that it offers long-term benefits for all age groups. "For modern, harried lifestyles focused on getting and spending, fitness experts say T'ai Chi, the ancient Chinese slow-moving exercise, can be an ideal way for anyone to stay fit." The article cited a 2007 National Health Interview Survey that stated that an estimated 2.3 million U. S. adults have done T'ai Chi in the past 12 months. "The practice is not perfect. T'ai Chi does not supply the cardiovascular component that we'd be looking for in a well-rounded routine," said Jessica Matthews, a San Diego,

California based exercise physiologist. "The exertion level while challenging, is not going to increase your heart rate."

www.reuters.com/article/2013/06/17/us-fitness-taichi-idUSBRE95G03E20130617

19. In May 18, 2013, Mayo Clinic had an article, "T'ai Chi: A gentle way to fight stress—T'ai Chi helps reduce stress and anxiety." And it also helps increase flexibility and balance. The article cites:

> "Tai chi is low impact and puts minimal stress on muscles and joints, making it generally safe for all ages and fitness levels ... You may also find tai chi appealing because it's inexpensive, requires no special equipment and can be done indoors or out, either alone or in a group."

www.mayoclinic.com/health/tai-chi/SA00087

(See article No. 15—September 28, 2012)

20. T'ai Chi Ireland: "Benefits of T'ai Chi." A very interesting description of the benefits to the physical body.

> The Body Alignments are opened ...
> Tai Chi strengthens the nerves and eases stress ...
> The blood is circulated without stress on the heart ...
> Tai Chi improves cardio-pulmonary function ...
> The lymph pump, hence the immune system,
>   is strengthened ...
> The synovial fluid is vitalised, bringing flexibility to
>   the joints ...
> The muscle tissue gains elasticity ...

The tendons are strengthened …
Tai Chi loosens the muscles and builds power …
Tai Chi creates balance in your life …

taichi-ireland.com/disciplines/benefits

21. "Breast Cancer Survivor Stays Fit with Tai Chi and Gi Gong," June 12, 2014, by Stacy Simonat, Stories of Hope for the American Cancer Society (www.cancer.org).

22. In February 3, 2015, (reviewed by David Zelman, MD, on June 10, 2013) in an article in Live Science titled "What is Tai Chi?" Elizabeth Palermo quotes Peter Wayne of Harvard Medical School as saying that tai chi is not just a physical activity:

> "[Tai chi] is a mind-body exercise that integrates slow, gentle movements, breathing and a variety of cognitive components, including focused attention, imagery and multi-tasking."

www.livescience.com/38063-tai-chi.html

23. In March 2015, an article from research done by Roger Jahnke, OMD, Linda Larkey, PhD, et al titled "A Comprehensive Review of Health Benefits of Qigong and Tai Chi," listed at the National Center for Biotechnology Information. This is extensive research from 2010 examining psychological and physiological benefits of *Qigong* and *Tai Chi* that is growing rapidly. It examines the evidence for achieving outcomes from substantial randomized controlled trials: physical function, falls and balance, quality of life,

self-efficacy, patient reported outcomes, psychological, immune function and inflammation.

www.ncbi.nlm.nih.gov/pmc/articles/PMC3085832

(See article No. 7—August 31, 2010)

24. In March 2015, reference is made by *Prevention Magazine*, "3 Reasons You Should Try Tai Chi And 3 ways to actually do it" from August 22, 2012 by Kristen Domonell. She states that adding *tai chi* to your life could help lower risk for developing dementia or Alzheimer's disease quoting from a new study in the *Journal of Alzheimer's Disease*. Researchers from the University of South Florida collaborated with Chinese researchers.

www.prevention.com/health/brain-health/health-benefits-tai-chi

25. In March 2015, an article by Mayo Clinic Staff refers to an article dated September 28, 2012 titled "Tai chi: A gentle way to fight stress—Tai chi helps reduce stress and anxiety." And it also helps increase flexibility and balance.

www.mayoclinic.org/healthy-lifestyles/stress-management/in-depth/tai-chi/art-20045184

(See article No. 15—September 28, 2012)

26. In March 2015 an article, "A guide to tai chi" in NHS Choices lists benefits: can help people aged 65 and over to reduce stress, to improve balance and general mobility, and increase muscle strength in the legs. Reviewed May 8, 2013.

www.nhs.uk/livewell/fitness/pages/taichi.aspx

27. In March 2015, an article on WebMD, "Health Benefits of Tai Chi and Qigong," states that "Many people who practice tai chi and qigong report heightened feelings of well-being along with a variety of other health benefits." These include: improved strength and better balance, reduced pain and stiffness, enhanced sleep, increased immunity to shingles, enhanced immune system, improved cardiovascular, respiratory, circulatory, lymphatic, and digestive functions; decreased risk of falling and reduced symptoms and improved function in people with fibromyalgia. This was reviewed by David Zelman, MD, June 10, 2013.

www.webmd.com/balance/guide/health-benefits-tai-chi-qigong

28. In March 2015, an article on MedicineNet.com, "Tai Chi," lists some documented benefits: balance and falling, improvement in self-confidence, strength and endurance, aerobic capacity, walking, fibromyalgia and stress. This was medically reviewed by a doctor on January 28, 2014.

www.medicinenet.com/tai_chi/page2.htm

29. In March 2015 extensive information by Vanderbilt University on "The Benefits of T'ai Chi." It covers history, motions, physical vs. mental benefits, joint and back problems, stress reduction, elderly, medical studies, cardiorespiratory functions, balance, flexibility and reduction of falls. Also included are Medical Studies on T'ai Chi: T'ai Chi and Cardiorespiratory Functions, T'ai Chi and Post-Stressor Recovery, T'ai Chi vs. Balance, Flexibility and More!, and T'ai Chi and The Reduction of Falls.

www.vanderbilt.edu/AnS/psychology/health_psychology/taichi2.htm

30. A list of articles found at www.networks.nhs.uk:

"Cardiac rehab," Feb. 21, 2011.

"Tai Chi for falls prevention," Feb. 21, 2011.

"Is mindfulness the answer to dealing with patient fears?," Feb. 25, 2011.

"Beat Alzheimer's and Dementia with Tai Chi," March 13, 2011.

"Tai Chi Improves Lung Function in COPD patients," March 13, 2011. (COPD: Chronic Obstructive Pulmonary Disease)

"Tai Chi Aids Osteoporosis recovery," April 28, 2011.

"Tai Chi and Chi-kung aid Obesity recovery," April 28, 2011.

"Tai Chi Helps Chronic Heart Failure Patients," May 3, 2011.

"Tai Chi May Improves Mental Health," May 4, 2011.

"Qigong and Tai Chi Research," May 10, 2011.

"Tai Chi at Kings College," June 15, 2011.

"Tai Chi alleviates Depression," Aug. 27, 2011.

"Tai Chi may improve Parkinson's symptoms: research," Feb. 13, 2012.

"Tai Chi reduces falls in people with failing eyesight," Feb. 28, 2012.

"New Study: Tai Chi Helps Improve Endurance, Balance, and Wellbeing of COPD Patients," Aug. 14, 2012.

"Breaking Medical Research: Finally, a Cure for the Common Cold?," Jan. 6, 2013.

"A Comprehensive Review of the Health Benefits of Qigong and Tai Chi," 1992 to 2000.

W.

Glossary

太极

Bubbling Spring: Known as *Hsueh* in Chinese, this refers to the sole of the foot, a key point in acupuncture. It is the focus of concentration in *T'ai Chi*. *T'ai Chi Ch'uan* teachers say that the *Chi* energy is drawn up through the soles of the feet (*Hsueh*) and distributed by the waist, which must be exceptionally pliable.

Chi: This word has many meanings in Chinese, but in *Ch'i Kung* it refers to the Vital Force, the intrinsic energy that flows through the meridian channels of the body. It is known as *ki* in Japanese, and can be referred to as *prana, shakti,* or *kundalini* in Indian languages. Also known as *Qi.*

Chih: This word also has many meanings. In *T'ai Chi Chih, Chih* means knowledge or knowing.

Ch'i Kung: The *Chi* can be separated into *Yin Chi* and *Yang Chi,* and the primary purpose of *Ch'i Kung* practices such as *T'ai Chi Chih* and *T'ai Chi Chuan* is to circulate and balance this *Chi. Ch'i Kung* is the science of the circulation of the *Chi.* Also known as *Qigong.*

Dantian: The *dantian* is translated as 'elixir field' or 'energy center.' *Dantians* are focal points for meditative techniques such as *Qigong* or *T'ai Chi* in Traditional Chinese Medicine. A *dantian* is a center of Qi or life-force energy.

Energy Sea: Around the lower *tan t'ien*, the spot two inches below the navel, there is believed to be a great reservoir of intrinsic energy, the Energy Sea, where the *Chi* is stored. It is from here that adepts in karate and aikido bring the energy with a great shout when they smash their fists through blocks of wood, for example.

Heart-Fire: The physical heart is the great *Yang* (positive) in the body, and corresponds to the sun in the heavens. The *Yang Chi* (energy from the heart level) is to be brought down for healing purposes to the spot two inches below the navel or to the soles of the feet. The *Chi* of the great *Yang*, the heart, is thus the *Heart-Fire*.

T'ai Chi Chih: A series of twenty separate movements that strongly circulates the *Chi*. Based on ancient principles, it was created by Justin Stone.

T'ai Chi Chuan: First of the martial arts, formerly called shadow boxing. Over a thousand years old in China, such disciplines as karate and aikido are thought to be derived from it. The classical form is a long dance of 108 movements, a true Moving Meditation.

T'ai Chi: Supreme Ultimate; a synonym of Tao.

Tao: Chinese word for Reality, seen by Chinese sages as a moving force, a flowing stream with which we should be in accord. It is often called Supreme Ultimate. Taoism is a philosophy that became a religion based on the concept of the all-embracing Tao.

Yin/Yang: Juxtaposition of any polarity, such as negative and positive. All Chinese cosmology is based on the interplay of these two types of energy, and the Moving Meditations attain their great benefits through balancing the circulated *Yin–Yang* energies. It is said by some scholars that the development of the computer was largely due to the *Yin–Yang* theory.

X.

Bibliography

太极

1. *Embrace Tiger, Return to Mountain*, by Al Chuang-liang Huang (Real People Press, Box F, Moab, Utah 84532, 1973), pp.169-70, 172-3.

2. *The Tao of T'ai-Chi Chuan, Way to Rejuvenation*, by Jou Tsung Hwa. (T'ai Chi Foundation, POB 828, Warwick, New York 10995, 1988).

3. *Yin and Yang*, by Huang Ti Nei Ching Su Wen.

4. *Written in Stone*, by Richard Cassaro, (Deeper Truth Books, LLC, New York City, 2011).

5. *From The Essence of T'ai Chi Ch'uan: A Literary Tradition*, translated and edited by Benjamin Pang Jeng Lo, Martin Inn, Robert Amacker, and Susan Foe, published by North Atlantic Books, 1979, by Benjamin Pang Jeng Lo, Martin Inn, Robert Amacker, and Susan Foe.

6. *The Swimming Dragon*, by T. K. Shih (Station Hill Press, Barrytown, New York 12507, 1989).

7. *Restoring Your Life Energy*, by Waysun Liao (Shambhala, Boston and London, 2012).

8. *T'ai Chi Chih! Joy Thru Movement*, by Justin F. Stone (Books and DVDs from Good Karma Publishing Company, Albuquerque, New Mexico).

9. *Taoist Ways to Transform Stress Into Vitality—The Inner Smile—Six Healing Sounds*, by Mantak Chia (Healing Tao Books, Huntington, New York, 1985).

10. *Healing Light of the Tao—Foundational Practices to Awaken Chi Energy*, by Mantak Chia (Destiny Books, Rochester, Vermont, 1993, 2008).

11. *Taoist Yoga, Alchemy and Immortality*, by Lu K'uan Yu (Red Wheel Weiser, Newbury Port, MA, 1970). A translation of the Secrets of Cultivating Essential Nature and Eternal Life by the Taoist Master Chao Pi Ch'en, born 1860.

12. *The Anatomy Coloring Book*, by Wynn Kapit and Lawrence M. Elson (Harper and Row Publishers, New York, 1977).

I must consider myself a pioneer who will contribute to the redefinition of aging. My chronological age and my biological age are two different things.

— Dr. Christiane Northrup

Y.

About
Virginia Harford

太极

A California native, Virginia now lives in San Miguel de Allende, Guanajuato, Mexico. Her background includes an Associate in Arts Degree in Recreational Leadership and a Bachelor of Science Degree in Physical Education from UCLA (University of California at Los Angeles).

She has had careers in business and education: as a dress buyer for a national retailer in Los Angeles and teaching ESL (English as a Second Language) in elementary through college levels. Virginia taught gentle exercises, breathing techniques and an accredited course of *T'ai Chi Chih* at Yavapai Retirement College in Arizona. She also instructed *Chi Kung* movements in Sedona, Arizona, San Diego, California, New Hampshire, Rio Caliente Spa near Guadalajara, Mexico, and San Miguel de Allende, Mexico, in 2013 and 2014. Virginia taught the first class of *T'ai Chi Chih* at the *T'ai Chih Chih* Center in Albuquerque when it opened in 1993.

Health and wellness have held a consistent and special interest for her, leading to Certification in Jin Shin Jyutsu (Acupressure), Reflexology, Rebirthing, Reiki and completing a year's program in Physical Fitness and Health Management from the University of California, San Diego at La Jolla. While in Europe, she attended the Sebastian Kneipp School, Bad Worishofen, Germany and obtained a Certificate in Introduction to Kneipp Physiotherapie and Spa Treatments. In Sedona, she studied gentle *Chi Kung* movements for longevity followed by becoming a certified teacher of *T'ai Chi Chih* in 1992. While living in New Mexico, she joined a group of *T'ai Chi* teachers meeting at Justin Stone's home for weekly practice. Justin was the creator of *T'ai Chi Chih.*

Virginia has visited many countries. She took a five-month trip around the world at one time, visiting Europe, India and the Orient. During three months, she visited many spa towns in Europe, then spent a month at an Indian ashram, and concluded with a return visit after twenty-five years to Kyoto, Japan. She also spent two weeks on a memorable trip to Peru. She continues to explore Mexico, her new home.

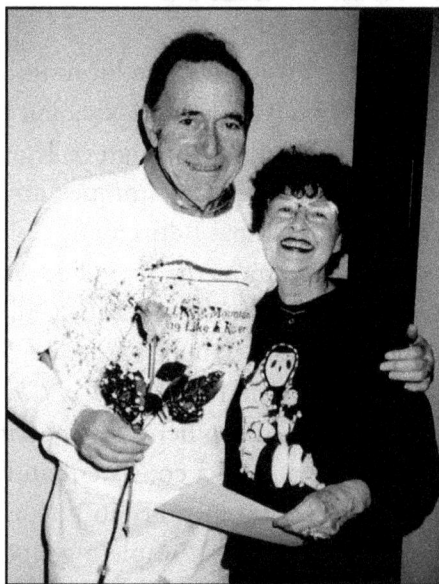

Virginia Harford receiving
her Seijaku Certificate
from Justin Stone in 1993.

www.ingramcontent.com/pod-product-compliance
Lightning Source LLC
Chambersburg PA
CBHW050351280326
41933CB00010BA/1418